THIS ISN'T THE LIFE I ORDERED...

THIS ISN'T THE LIFE I ORDERED...

Setting Sail When Your Relationship Fails.

JENNIFFER WEIGEL

Published by Waterfront Press 2015
www.waterfrontdigitalpress.com

ISBN: 978-1-941768-92-1 ebook
ISBN: 978-1-941768-93-8 print edition

TABLE OF CONTENTS

Foreward vii

Acknowledgments xi

Chapter 1   Tale as Old as Time 1
Chapter 2   Floating with the Tide 27
Chapter 3   Love Your Shadow 34
Chapter 4   Back in the Saddle 51
Chapter 5   Kicked Out of Heaven 70
Chapter 6   Wisdom from an $800 Pair of shoes 96
Chapter 7   Sometimes We Need to Get Drunk on
             a Wayne-Anita Cocktail 105
Chapter 8   Thank you, Jesus 124
Chapter 9   Some Things Can't be Fixed with a
             Bag of Ice 135
Chapter 10   Tale of Two Theories 148
Chapter 11   Fear is Like a Beach Ball 168
Chapter 12   You Gotta Fix Yourself Before
             You Can Fix the World 176
Chapter 13   John of God 198
Chapter 14   Tears in my Tiramisu 235
Chapter 15   I love you. I'm sorry. Forgive me. Thank you. 253
Chapter 16   Slow Down and Enjoy the View 269

FOREWARD

By Caroline Myss

I was thrilled to read Jenniffer's new book on relationships, not only because she is an entertaining writer, but because she uses her skillful talent as a writer to slip in much needed social wisdom about the challenges we are confronting in the arena of the heart.

I have long been fascinated with the evolution of the Marriage Archetype; more specifically, how we as individuals have inadvertently outgrown the parameters of this long-standing band of commitment. Over the course of the past five or six decades, our emphasis on personal growth, individualism, self-help, and empowerment workshops have resulted in awakening an appetite for, well, putting our own needs front and center in our lives. Prior to the days of these personal options, such an emphasis on oneself would have been considered an act of unparalleled selfishness. Today the preface "self" is now capitalized and it implies an inner being: The Inner Self. We consider the Inner Self to be an actual entity, a type of "significant inner other" to whom we look for inner guidance.

Our Inner Self has the first and last word when it comes to directing our intimate lives. It gives us permission to do what was considered socially, morally, and sexually unthinkable decades ago. In fact, our Inner Self can talk us into spending sprees the likes of which would be considered ridiculously irresponsible prior to this age of the "Self". Now, all we have to do is rely upon our Inner Self to come up with a few wounds from previous relationships to explain unacceptable behavioral patterns and we are, more or less, off the hook. I know countless stories of couples whose relationships came to a close because one or the other received guidance from their Inner Self instructing them to go on walk-abouts because they needed to find themselves. Others felt that their Inner Self was telling them that they were unhappy and unfulfilled in their relationship and had to move on.

Still others found that while they wanted to be in a relationship, each time the relationship approached the commitment borderline, their Inner Self would hit a panic button. The common issue was "space". That is, the Inner Self requires a great deal of space and personal time and attention in which to thrive; thus, while the person longs for a relationship and the intimacy that goes along with forming such a bond, what ever do they do about this need their Inner Self has for its own space, time, privacy, and independence?

It would appear that the emergence of the Inner Self and its unique values are in direct collision with the long-standing values of the Marriage Archetype. I see that as one of the leading challenges of contemporary relationships. And from that one major challenge come all the others. Essentially, the solid values once represented by traditional marriage – such as the vow understood to be sacred – no longer have the same clout or meaning. The problem is we have yet to replace any of those solid values with anything that can stand up to a windy day, much less survive a serious commitment.

The truth is we have lost faith in our capacity to go the distance with anything, from jobs to the banks hanging together to our nation surviving. Is it any wonder that people do not trust the longevity of the relationship commitment? Honestly and integrity have evaporated as social and moral values, so much so that couples need to seek out a third party such as a marriage counselor in order to say one honest sentence to their spouse. How frightening is that? Spouses sleep with each other, have their meals together, have children together, pay their bills together and require a third party in order to navigate an honest sentence, What does that tell you about their ability to model integrity for their children? Think about that.

Relationships are in a crisis for so many reasons, not the least of which is that the values required to make relationships work are contrary to the values of the Inner Self, which is fundamentally "me" centered. The Inner Self should be a type of temporary state of consciousness, a psychological boat one takes across the river of transformation. You have to get off on the other side as a whole person who is capable of loving and caring for the "other" without fearing that you will lose yourself in the process. Jenniffer's book only enforced my position all the more – and I personally thank her for that.

The stories in Jenniffer's books are statements of our time. She has captured the crisis with precision because she also rode the storm of a marriage and a divorce. Jenniffer is one of those reporters who has a knack for writing not only about something she knows, but something she has lived – and in many ways, is still living.

This is a book for every one who has ever gone near the fires of a personal relationship. It's wonderful when wisdom is wrapped up in great writing.

Caroline Myss
Oak Park July 2014

ACKNOWLEDGMENTS

I've always thought the acknowledgments in a book are kind of like watching the Oscars - they can be way too long and nobody wants to hear Ang Lee thank his lawyer. So let's make this short and sweet:

This book is dedicated to my son Britt who inspires me to be the best I can be. To Bill Gladstone and Jack Jennings who both believed in my writing since my first book "Stay Tuned". To those authors, healers and friends who allowed me to use their wisdom - Billy Corgan, Amy Dickinson, Lisa Dietlin, Wayne Dyer, Anne Emerson, Bela Gandhi, Anita Moorjani, Sara Morrison, Caroline Myss, Dr. Mary Neal, David Prete, Therese Rowley, John St. Augustine, Gail Thackray and John of God.

To Megan Robinson for the excellent book cover photo (www.megan-magill.com) and to the slew of friends who have been there for me through this transition - you know who you are and I couldn't have done this work on myself without you.

And for anyone who struggles with finding their path or true calling. I can relate, so shoot me an email if this book inspires you – www.jenweigel.com

Love yourself – don't leave yourself.

CHAPTER ONE
TALE AS OLD AS TIME

Facebook Status:

Heard on Michigan Avenue: "Look at you! If we were married, I'd be banging you every day."

"No Danny, if we were married, we wouldn't be having sex, because that's what happens to married people."

⚜ ⚜ ⚜

"We have this idea of what love is that's based on the myths that we see in pop culture. From women's magazines, to movies, to pop songs, an unrealistic standard is perpetuated that's impossible to achieve. We don't need to change our partners; we need to change our way of thinking." – Tim Ray, author of the book "101 Relationship Myths: How to Stop Them From Sabotaging Your Happiness."

⚜ ⚜ ⚜

"Don't get divorced unless your husband is a heroin addict or beats the shit out of you," my friend said to me at a book club gathering. My second book had been released and she was hosting an event at her home. "I don't even have kids and my divorce was hell," she added. "Avoid it at all costs. Go to counseling."

"We've been to counseling for five years – both together and separately," I said.

"It is like a death," she said. "Make sure you're absolutely positive before you do this."

Is anyone ever absolutely positive about a divorce? If I stayed in the marriage, I'd be unhappy, If I left,

I'd be unhappy. I knew either way I'd be screwed.

"Did he cheat?" She asked.

"No."

"Did you?"

"No."

"Then what is it?"

I don't know!

"Sometimes love isn't enough and people change," I said. "We're roommates instead of partners. It's been like this for a long time."

When you decide to end a marriage and there is no huge scandal, affair or addiction to blame for the split, people get pissed off. What used to seem like similar paths now felt like a distant memory. I married a good man. He married a good woman. And when you no longer bring out the best in each other, maybe you shouldn't stay married?

But that's not necessarily going to satisfy your girlfriends, mother or party guests. They want a thing/person/phobia to blame. If you don't provide this, they are confused.

"Why not just live separate lives and stick together for your son?" one woman suggested. "Just have different bedrooms and go your own way and he can go his way."

I know lots of people who do this, actually. You may have seen them at parent teacher conferences. They sit together growling under their breath but pretend everything is great; and you suspect that he's screwing his co-worker and she's banging the soccer coach. (But at least they all get to have the holidays together.)

And I get it. It's a hell of a lot easier to just live in different ends of the house, keep all your stuff and stay in your kids' daily lives.

I didn't want to live separately from my spouse. I wanted a partner. Someone to share things with and enjoy on a daily basis. Not somebody to nag and argue with whenever we opened our mouths.

How did we get here?

"Where's your husband?" The best friend of my book club hostess asked me. She'd met him at a party the previous Christmas.

I didn't even know how to tell my own family that my 13-year-marriage was crumbling, let alone a woman I'd met casually at a cookie exchange. But the faking it part was becoming exhausting.

It's just not the right time.

Is there ever a right time to announce a divorce?

"I'm putting my house on the market and we are separated," I blurted out.

There were several gasps in the room. A few of those in attendance had also met my husband. All of them loved us as a couple (and this was just based on my two books, not from having us over for cookouts or anything.)

As I worked my way through the room later that night I overheard two of the mothers chatting. They were probably in their late 60's. One leaned in to the other and said, "People today just don't try anymore. They don't honor their vows. It's such a shame."

I almost dropped my wine glass.

Nobody gets married with the hope that one day you'll be calling a lawyer and fighting over who gets the oriental rugs. I married my best friend when I was 27. During our tenure together we buried three of our four parents, had a child and rehabbed a house. I thought if we could make it through all of that we could get through anything.

"The plan was to grow old and change each others' diapers when we could no longer make it to the toilet. Period!" I said to the woman hosting the book party.

I started to notice things shift in my marriage after our son was born. I'd somehow turned into my husband's mother and he had become my child – a dynamic we discovered and both admitted to in therapy.

I already had one child and didn't want another.

And nobody wants to sleep with their mother.

"Did you hear about Molly?" One of the women said. "She reconnected with her ex-boyfriend from high school on Facebook, and now they're both getting divorced and getting back together."

Oh sweet Jesus.

"I told her she needs to go to therapy but she's already filing for divorce," she continued.

I knew one couple that went to therapy for two sessions before calling it quits.

Really? Two sessions with a shrink is all you'll give your 15-year marriage?

Turns out, she'd started having an affair and left her husband for that other man. They are now happily married and basically the Brady Bunch; but I can't help but wonder if it will last, considering how it began. But hell, maybe she'll prove me wrong and that can be the subject of my next book: "How to screw your married neighbor when you're married and make it last a lifetime."

My version looks a little different. I feel that if you have had kids with someone, you have to go to therapy with your spouse at least a dozen times – or once a month for a year – before you jump ship. Why a whole year? Because even if there's an affair, once the endorphins wear off, you're left with the same problems you had in your previous relationship. You start looking at your ex and thinking, "Maybe he wasn't so bad after all?" But you're already divorced. Still, you decide to "date" your ex and take the whole broken, now reunited family on vacation, which can totally screw up your kids.

I know this only because I lived it. My parents got divorced when I was four, then started dating again when I was five. The man my mom often referred to as "that son-of-a-bitch" was taking all of us to the Wisconsin Dells. It was a very confusing time. Don't do this.

I beg you.

Then there was the friend who told me that a priest was going to fix all her problems because "therapy is for crazy people."

I couldn't help but laugh at the thought that they were putting their marriage in the hands of someone who allegedly has never had sex (with a woman at least?) or been married.

I've had good therapists and I've had bad ones. How do you know the difference? If you've been seeing a therapist for more than four visits and you don't feel you've made any progress, you don't have the right therapist. Do you want suggestions or do you just need to be heard? It all depends on your issues of course, but be picky when choosing your therapist. It's your time and your money, so know what you're looking for and shop around. Your mental health depends on it.

When I was about 10 my parents decided that my brother and I needed to see a therapist after they each had remarried other people. I have these distinct memories of a therapist sitting in a chair taking notes and nodding their head, saying one simple phrase over and over again: "How did that make you *feel*?"

I felt like the therapist didn't really care how I felt but was asking the question because they were getting paid. How did I feel? *I want to go home and watch Scooby Doo now, please.*

When I was in my twenties, I thought I'd give therapy a try again after an emotional breakup with a boyfriend. I actually found someone who was a little more proactive. We established goals and she would give me feedback. It was much more encouraging.

"Psychotherapy today is not your parent's therapy," one of the women from the book club crowd said. "People feel they don't have the time or the money to waste dwelling on their childhoods." She would know because she's a therapist.

After I got married, I had a life coach who also did individual therapy sessions. He then became my therapist and my husband's life coach. Eventually, he took on the task of being our couples' therapist. (I have trouble establishing boundaries.)

But after five years we weren't making much progress in couple's therapy.

"You've been at this way too long to not be getting results," my one therapist friend insisted.

But I like our counselor so much as a person!

"Just because you like someone doesn't mean they should be your therapist," she said.

What I had on my hands was a well-intentioned life coach who cared deeply for my well being and wanted to see me through this bump in the road, but had no degree for therapy training.

"If you were remodeling a kitchen for five years and you still didn't have the kitchen you wanted, you'd either fire your architect or give up on the damn kitchen," my therapist friend pointed out.

Maybe she has a point.

When we went to our first session with a new couple's therapist, we quickly learned within minutes that our usual m.o. wasn't going to fly.

"This is not the place to re-enact your fights. And absolutely no swearing in this office is allowed," she said.

No fucking swearing?

We learned more in one session about our issues than we had with our previous therapist over a year's time. Not only did she point out our patterns, she gave us tools to communicate with each other. While it didn't save our marriage, it gave us a foundation that helped us through the divorce.

"My ex never went to therapy with me," the woman hosting the book party confessed. "I had to drag him the first time, and he quit after one session because he said he felt ganged up on.'"

The truth about therapy is that you really have to look under the hood and tattle on yourself. I get why people don't like to go because nobody likes to admit they're flawed.

"Thank God I had Alan during my divorce," one of the women said as she sipped her wine. Alan was a man from her past. They reconnected when her marriage was on the rocks and started a whirlwind affair while she was going through couples' therapy.

For the record, I don't recommend this either.

You can't look at your wounds and try to save your marriage when you're getting laid in the back of a LandRover after carpooling the kids to school.

So I amend my earlier rule: if someone is having sex with a person who is NOT their spouse during couples' therapy, the therapy for any amount of time (especially for a year) is a waste of time and money.

But that's the only exception.

"Are you officially separated now?" one of the women asked me.

The NEW way of separating (according to some article I read in the New York Times) is having your kid(s) stay in the house while the parents come and go. This way, the children aren't disrupted by the back-and-forth while you give your marriage mouth-to-mouth.

Of course, this method ain't cheap.

"I found an apartment online, and we're going to take turns going between our house and the apartment while Britt stays in the house," I said.

Every three days, Britt just thought Mommy and Daddy kept getting on airplanes and taking lots of trips because we always had roll-on luggage.

Looking back on this experience, I think it was a really bad idea. You can't get a sense for being divorced by sharing two residences. You both have your belongings at each place, so you're roommates in two homes instead of one, (but hey – who am I to argue with the New York Times?)

What this experiment did show me, however, is the absolute misery that comes from wanting to be with your child when you cannot. This "forced exile" was, by far, the most important step toward my soon-to- be divorce. It showed me what it would really be like if we ended our marriage. And despite my best efforts, those lonely nights in a tiny apartment can't be soothed with HBO and a cosmo.

"Nobody will ever say you took this divorce lightly," one of the women said, reaching for an appetizer. "I've never seen someone try so hard to make something work."

"But how long do you try until you give up?" I asked. "Is five years of therapy enough? Six? Eight? When do you say, 'it's time to go our separate ways?'"

My parents were so angry with each other after their divorce they couldn't be in the same room without raising their voices – until I was 18. People would always ask me if I wanted them to get back together, and I'd always say, "I don't want them in the same zip code!!"

My husband's parents were married to each other for over thirty years. But just because you stay married doesn't mean you'll be a shining example to your children of what a relationship should look like.

"We are really trying to do this differently," I said. We weren't always successful, but the fact that it was a priority helped me sleep at night.

"My parents still hate each other," one woman said. "It makes the holidays a total nightmare because we have to split up the day with each of them. It's exhausting."

I remember the first time my parents sat at a table and didn't scream at each other. I was 19 and my brother was 20. We had an event at college and both parents decided to show up at the same time. We thought it might "kill two birds with one stone" if we had breakfast as a family for the first time since 1976. It was awkward but we survived. And each time they were together after that, things got a bit less tense. By the time Dad married his third wife Vicki, my Mom was invited over for the holidays.

"The reason your mom and I get along is because there was a buffer wife," Vicki would joke, referring to wife number two whom everybody hated.

I try to imagine Britt as a young adult and then fantasize that his father and I are there for him, getting along as a family.

Maybe we'll be at his college "parent's weekend," sitting in a restaurant, having dinner, just the three of us. Britt will have my laugh and his father's keen sense of humor; and he'll lean in to the two of us and say, "I'm so glad you two are here with me – together."

And his father and I will look at each other and smile, knowing that we tried everything. Our contract expired as husband and wife, but it will never expire as his parents.

"My ex is a drunk and he gets extremely violent around my kids," one woman in the back of the book party said. "I vowed until 'death do us part' but I can't put my babies in danger," she continued, holding back tears. "He won't cooperate with the lawyers so my kids are in this limbo. It's awful. I've been fighting for two years."

Here's something that many adults seem to forget in the emotional throws of a divorce: When you don't respond to lawyers and continue to fight with a spouse who wants a divorce, the only one who loses is you (by paying a shitload of money to your lawyers) and your kids (who learn that this is how you're supposed to behave when things don't go your way).

Another woman approached me and spoke of a marriage gone cold. There was no big affair or horrible addiction – just apathy.

"I get the feeling he hates himself, and so he takes it out on me and the kids," she said. "He's been out of work for years and he's really depressed. I have two jobs so we can keep our house."

"Is he getting help?" I asked.

"He's gone to therapy a couple of times," she said.

"How long has it been like this?" I asked.

"Five years," she said.

Life is too short to be faced with five years of apathy.

"Even he admitted that I've been the only one working on this marriage for the last five years," she said. "I'm so tired I can't even see straight."

I then launched into my theory of how contracts expire. I feel (and I've been in four of my parents' weddings, so I'm a bit of an expert) that just because we say "I do" doesn't mean we have to stick around when things get toxic or we no longer celebrate being married to our spouse. People are meant to be in our lives at different stages of our journey. We aren't meant to stay anywhere for an eternity. If the dynamics change in the relationship, and you've really tried everything to make it work, you are allowed to renegotiate the contract. And if both parties don't agree on the terms, it's time to end the contract altogether.

"I feel like my mom and dad were meant to get married and have kids because my brother and I were supposed to be born. But after that, they shouldn't have stayed together as long as they did because all they did was fight," I said.

I could see the heaviness in this woman's eyes lighten with my words.

"My sister told me there's a town in Ireland where every married couple is given the chance to reassess their marriage every seven years," said one of the women. "The whole town comes together at that point, and the family and friends look at the union, and everyone votes on whether they should stay married or go their separate ways. There is no big drama about it either."

I'm moving to Ireland.

"There is no doubt that my children were supposed to be born," said the woman whose husband was a drinker. "But they deserve better than this."

"And so do you," I said. "And just because a marriage ends, that doesn't mean it was a failure. It was a gift because you had your children. You have to look at the good that came from it rather than focus on the fact that it didn't last for a lifetime. I mean, if we think about how the whole 'I do' thing got started a couple thousand years ago, women were the property of men. The whole thing was a contract between families. And people were dying when they were 34."

"I just don't know what I did wrong," one of the women said, trying not to sob.

"Who says you did anything wrong?!" I yelled.

There is actually a book called "Confessions of a Recovering Stupid Male". I know this because I interviewed the author. And I asked him what mistake women continue to make in relationships, and his answer surprised me.

"They don't believe in themselves. The number one reason why women stay in relationships other than for financial reasons is that they have low self esteem. They believe they aren't powerful or that they aren't whole if they aren't with a man. A year ago the Dalai Lama said the fate of the planet rests on the western woman. You're not going to see that on the front pages of the papers, but you should because we need to have that feminine energy. Women don't realize how powerful they are or how much they matter, whether they're with or without a man."

⚜   ⚜   ⚜

A couple weeks later, I was talking on television about a column I'd written about divorce.

"Sometimes contracts expire," I said.

When I returned to my desk, I found the following email:

"I just listened to your conversation on TV regarding couples – "Sometimes Contracts Expire". Are you kidding me? Options expire. Land contracts expire. God made marriage a lifetime contract. Get a life. Jack."

I immediately wrote back:

"Hey Jack,
Sometimes people aren't meant to stay married. You mean to tell me if a husband is beating the crap out of his wife, or a drunk who never comes home, or hits his kids ... these people are supposed to be in a lifetime contract? That's not what happened in my marriage, but I know people who are in these situations. They stay because of a vow and they do irreparable damage to their children. People make mistakes and it's okay to walk away despite making a VOW. I respectfully will COMPLETELY disagree with you."

Within minutes, he responded,

"It's because of liberals like you that today's generation finds it easy to walk away from a marriage rather than work out the difficulties. Please do not reply, I don't like conversing with idiots. Jack."

Liberals like me?

I was about to unleash a string of obscenities that would have made my Dad proud, until he followed with this:

"Your father would be rolling in his grave."

Now you claim to know my Dad?

I almost wrote the sentence, "Do you know how many times my Dad got married?" but I was frozen in place by his next comment.

"No wonder you're getting divorced," he added.

Ouch.

Still fuming from my email exchange with a mother-fucking idiot, I saw another email pop up on my screen. It was from my realtor.

"You may need to think about lowering the price of your house," she said. "Unless you want to just hold onto it until spring and put it back on the market after the holidays."

Both my husband and I thought we priced our house to sell. It had been shown more times than any other house they had listed. Yet there hadn't been one offer.

"What gives?" I said when I called my friend, intuitive Therese Rowley, to tell her about my frustrating day.

"You won't get an offer until you let go of the house and make a clear decision," she said.

"What do you mean?"

"You're in limbo," she said. "So nothing is going to land until you are clear about your plans. There is a fog of uncertainty around you. Until you are clear about your next steps, a buyer won't find your house."

"Damn you psychics!" I joked.

"I'm not a psychic. I'm an intuitive," she laughed. "There's a difference."

Therese was right. While I was separated, neither of us had filed for divorce. We were still going to therapy but it didn't seem to be helping. And for a while we each wanted to find a way where one of us could keep the house. First, he was going to buy me out. Then, I was going to buy him out. It had become a sore subject all around because we both felt like we'd put everything we had into this place.

Which we had...

"I was supposed to have my ashes sprinkled in the backyard when I died," I said.

"It's just a house," Therese said. "You can't take it with you."

❧ ❧ ❧

Before moving to the burbs, my husband and I had always wanted to be city dwellers. We had plans to move out of our condo and into a townhouse, until things took a sharp left turn – my Dad died, then his mom died, and we found ourselves wondering what life would be like with a yard and a parking space.

So one night, I decided to pray to my dead Dad. While it seemed sort of silly to be yapping at the ceiling, bestselling author and medium James Van Praagh told me when I interviewed him that we should always talk to our dead loved ones like they're in the next room. "They can hear you," he insisted. "They will give you signs and signals."

I'd now made it a habit to talk to the air with requests for Dad, as if he had nothing better to do.

"OK Dad, I think I want to move to Evanston, but I'm not sure if I should look up there, so can you give me a sign?" I said, sort of laughing at my own request. "Thanks. Hope you're well."

The following morning, I woke up to an email in my inbox from a realtor I hadn't heard from in two years. She'd sent me a listing of a house in the suburbs.

This has to be a mistake!

I picked up the phone and called her immediately.

"Hi Julie, it's Jen Weigel," I said.

"Hi Jen, how are you?" she asked, sounding surprised.

"I'm great. Just looking at this email you sent me about a listing. Any reason you sent this my way?" I asked.

There was a long pause, followed by,

"I didn't send you an email."

Cue Twilight Zone soundtrack.

"I'm looking at it right here," I said.

"Send it back to me," she said. "I have no idea how that got to you."

I sent her back the email.

"That is so weird. Are you even looking?" She asked.

"I think I am NOW!" I said.

I made an appointment to go and look at this home. I was somehow convinced that my Dad was sending me signs from the grave that this was the house of my dreams (even though it was totally out of my price range) and everything else would fall into place.

When I arrived, I couldn't believe my eyes because the house was kind of a dump.

"Not a lot of curb appeal," I said.

We walked inside, and it wasn't much better.

What are you trying to pull here, Dad? This house sucks.

As I sat out front wondering what kind of practical joke my Dad was up to from beyond, the realtor said, "You know, there is this foreclosure around the corner that I think I need to show you."

"What street is it on?" I asked.

"Grant," she said.

Grant? I GREW UP on Grant.

As we pulled up to this gorgeous Tudor home, I was in awe. It seemed like a castle. It had been abandoned for six months, so the yard was a bit overgrown; but it had incredible bones, and shockingly, it was in our price range.

"What happened?" I asked. This was years before foreclosures were the norm. I'd never even heard of a foreclosure, let alone understood how it works.

"The husband had some bad investment deals and over-borrowed on the house, I guess," she said. "They got divorced."

A lawyer once told me, "Someone else's tragedy could lead to your next opportunity." (Leave it to a lawyer to come up with that one.)

We made an offer on it that night, but quickly learned several others had outbid us.

"Oh well," I said. "I guess it wasn't meant to be."

But later that night, we got the call.

"I can't believe this, but you got the house!" My realtor said, practically yelling through the phone.

"How is that possible?" I asked.

"The other offers were higher, but you had the cleanest offer," she said. "Everyone else had a sales contingency to deal with. You guys could move right in and close right away so they picked you."

Our excitement turned to panic when we realized we had to renovate a four-bedroom house. This place needed new plumbing, new electric, a new kitchen. You name it, it needed it. But that's why the price was right. Our new life was unfolding and we were ready to take it on, head first.

That Christmas Eve, just a few days before our closing, we drove by our soon-to-be new house and sat in the driveway. The snow was falling as Nat King Cole's "A Christmas Song" played on the radio. We stared in disbelief at the beautiful home that was going to be ours. I suddenly felt like such a grown-up. The excitement of what was ahead filled me up like the snow covering the sidewalk.

"I can't believe it," my husband said, holding my hand.

"We are going to live here the rest of our lives," I said.

⚜ ⚜ ⚜

Back to the future: I was being talked off the ledge by Therese. The house of my dreams would one day be inhabited by strangers who wouldn't appreciate all we'd done and there was nothing I could do about it.

"That house was meant to be mine," I said.

"You can create a loving home for you and Britt anywhere," she said. "Until you decide to let this go, nobody will make an offer. You have to let go of the house."

My contract with my beautiful house had expired.

⚜ ⚜ ⚜

The following day, my husband and I had the unpleasant conversation of what we realistically should do to move forward. We both admitted that it didn't make financial sense for either of us to keep the house. We would lower the price one more time before the holidays and if nothing happened, we'd take it off the market until the spring.

One week after we lowered the price and "let go" of the house, we got an offer. (In a down market and a week before Thanksgiving, mind you!) We went from thinking we'd have a few months to get organized, to needing a place to move the Monday after Christmas.

Shit!

"I told you," Therese said.

My house search went into high gear. My husband decided to take the "separation apartment" after the move, so he was set. I looked high and low, but apparently, Thanksgiving isn't the best season to find your "Plan B" house.

Then one day my mother came over when I was packing boxes.

"Your father must be upset with me or something," she said.

My parents got divorced in 1975, dated again in 1976, and were done for good in 1977.

"My dead father is upset with you?" I asked.

"Well, he always sends me signs in the form of a black squirrel, and I haven't seen one in so long," she said. "I'm really getting upset."

Another thing that James Van Praagh told me is that our loved ones will show up in in the form of wildlife. For me, Dad seems to show up as a cardinal; for my Mom, it's a black squirrel.

"I pray to him to help you," she said. "I just wish I could make it easier for you, sweetie."

No mom wants to see her child in pain.

"I need to go for a run," I said. "Can you watch Britt so I can clear my head?" I asked.

Running had been my salvation. I had been doing it almost daily, like a meditation. I had a route that I took that never changed: three miles, less than thirty minutes, start to finish.

But as I went outside, I found myself taking a left turn rather than my usual right.

Where are you going, Jen?

I had no idea why I went a different direction. I ran for about a mile and there it was – a black squirrel staring at me from a nearby tree. I never see black squirrels.

It's just a coincidence.

I made another right and was amazed when a second black squirrel popped out of yet another tree. Black squirrels are not that common in my area. One was unusual enough, but two was almost unheard of.

Mom is gonna be pissed I'm getting all the squirrel love!

Not two minutes later I turned a corner, and I was startled to see a third black squirrel. It was lifting its tail making horrible noises like it was going to attack something. The sight and the sounds made me stop in my tracks.

"What!" I yelled, slightly worried that I was now screaming at a rat with a tail up in a tree.

I turned in the direction where the squirrel was looking, and right in front him was a house for sale with a sign that read "Open today 12-2".

I thought I'd seen every house on realtor.com, but this one did not look familiar. It was really small but charming enough where I wanted to look inside.

When I got home, I told my mom about the squirrels.

"I'm going to look at that house now because of it. I probably wouldn't have stopped if you hadn't mentioned the squirrels in the first place. So thank you," I said.

"He *is* listening," Mom said, looking at the sky.

I took Britt with me to look at it a couple hours later. When we pulled up, one of those damn black squirrels was in the tree.

OK, OK. I'm here, aren't I?!

"I like this house Mommy," Britt said as we parked. He'd been with me on several open house outings, although he didn't really know why.

We walked inside. It was an old one-story farmhouse from the late 1800's, complete with crooked floors and tiny rooms, but it felt cozy to me.

"Let's look at the yard, Mom," said Britt.

We walked through the long screened porch to a yard that was surprisingly bigger than ours. I took a deep breath. I tried to picture myself staring at the sky and listening to the trees blow in the wind as I swung in a hammock. I looked at the landscaping and saw beautiful flowers. The woman who lived there loved her garden, just like me.

And that's when I decided that house would be mine.

"They don't have any toys here, Mom," Britt said, looking at the yard.

"I think that's because they don't have any kids," I explained.

"That's so sad," Britt said, genuinely concerned. He was four going on 35.

As we walked through the house to leave, Britt went to the realtor and said, "Thank you. I really like your house!"

She looked at him surprised and said, "You're welcome young man."

I made an offer when I got home. Three days later, the house was ours.

The night I received the news that I'd gotten the house, I went upstairs and looked at Britt sleeping. While I was happy to have a place for us to go, I felt like such a failure. By moving into a tiny little place, I was admitting that everything I'd worked for – my marriage and my life in this beautifully renovated home – was now lost. I didn't want Britt to feel this loss, too. How would I tell him that he has to pack up all his toys and leave the only house he's ever known?

"Oh, and by the way kiddo – the new house is about one third the size of your old one, and you and mommy will be sharing a bathroom."

Sometimes things just don't turn out the way you planned.

And when life gives you lemons, you need to make a lemon drop martini.

I went downstairs to the kitchen and paused as I stood before the fridge. We had several magnets strewn about – all different snapshots of our life reminding me of happier times. One picture of the three of us playing on the bed was front and center. Looking at it felt like a punch in the gut. I was suddenly overwhelmed by this colossal disappointment. Disappointment in myself. Disappointment in my marriage. Disappointment in my life and how things didn't go as planned.

I'm so sorry, Britt.

I went into the family room and decided to put in a movie. Inside the DVD player was *Beauty and the Beast,* which had become one of Britt's favorites. As I put it away, I remembered the last time Britt and I had been watching it together. My husband came in the door with his luggage and walked into the family room. It was my turn to head to the apartment, but I sat there watching my son gaze as Beauty and the Beast danced in the large ballroom.

"What's everyone watching?" he asked.

Britt looked at the two of us, pointed to the area in front of the TV and barked an order.

"Dance!"

Dance?

We both let out a nervous laugh, hoping the order would dissolve into thin air. Then Britt grabbed both of our hands and put them together. He was only four and he wanted his mommy and daddy to dance.

"Dance!" he said again. He was not going to take "No" for an answer.

My husband and I looked at each other, and the next thing I knew, I was in his arms as we rocked from side to side. The man who had been such a stranger lately was now holding me in his arms. We had shared the last 15 years together. Somehow, all the fighting and frustration that had been part of our daily grind was nowhere in sight. I tried to hide that I was wiping away tears.

"Tale as old as time, song as old as rhyme, Beauty and the Beast ..."

My nose rested on my husband's neck. I could smell his skin as we slipped into a familiar rhythm that felt so…..natural. He was never big on dancing. Swaying side to side was the only dance he would do willingly. We had done this so many times before – but never with the knowledge that this could very well be the last time we were partners.

I saw Britt alternate between watching the TV, and watching us. I tried not to cry in front of him, but there had been so many tears over the last few months this goal was getting harder to accomplish. I couldn't tell if my husband was crying as well. I do know that he held me tight, and I held him back.

If only it were this easy.

That was our last dance.

❖ ❖ ❖

Chapter Two
Floating with the Tide

Facebook Status:

"Is there school tomorrow?" Britt asked. "Yes," I said. "Oh man. I wish I could be like Sponge Bob and just work at the Crusty Crab," he replied.

⚜ ⚜ ⚜

"The sign of a truly successful negotiation is when both sides are pissed off," a lawyer told me.

My husband and I were moving forward with the divorce and it was time to divide 15 years worth of stuff.

For the most part we had been pretty civil to each other during the process, but we'd started bickering about art.

"Buy your own paintings," my mom said. "It's not worth the stress."

We'd agreed to sell most of our furniture on Craigslist to the highest bidder since we were both going to substantially scale down our living arrangements. Whatever we couldn't sell was going to the Salvation Army.

From towels to books, every item brought up a memory. Putting these into boxes and knowing I'd never see them again was taking an emotional toll. I picked up a heavy handmade blanket. It had been knitted by my husband's grandmother and neither of us wanted to take it with us.

I wonder if the new owner will appreciate it?

On top of the pain that came with packing up my life, I was also panicking about work. While I continued to do book talks and write, I didn't have a steady paycheck and nothing was on the horizon.

I called my agent to let him know I was back on the broadcast market.

"Put my hat in the ring for anything," I said.

"Anything?" He asked. He'd reached out to me in the past when reporting jobs were available.

But several years earlier I'd made such a big deal about leaving my job as a TV reporter to follow my dream of telling stories that didn't involve fires and hit-and-run accidents. I'm sure he thought he wasn't hearing me correctly.

"Yes," I said, feeling defeated.

Two weeks later, he called with a job.

"They're looking for a traffic reporter for the mornings on Oldies," he said.

Traffic reporter?

I'd started my broadcasting career as a traffic reporter. I was always tired and the money was crappy. Getting up at 3 a.m. to talk about the outbound Kennedy to O'Hare was my version of job hell.

Been there, done that.

"I did that job in '97," I said, pouting. "There's nothing else?"

"Not at the moment," he said.

The traffic job did have health insurance; but it felt like I'd be taking several steps back rather than moving forward.

"Let's keep looking," I said.

What gives, universe? That's the best you've got?

I'd been trying to trust that there was some sort of master plan with my career search, but I was starting to lose faith. All the gurus that I'd interviewed over the years had given me plenty of wisdom; so far, I was having trouble following their advice.

I remembered don Miguel Ruiz who wrote "The Four Agreements" telling me if you want something to land in your world, you have to be "the wide open field."

"Think of a plane landing on a runway. It's not going to land where there is chaos. You have to be the wide open runway. Calm and open. Then something will find you."

He also said you have to plant the seeds and nurture the garden, and then at some point you have to sit back and let the plants grow.

"You can't pull on the stalks to make them grow faster," he said.

You can't?

The next night I was doing my live show called "Wednesdays With Weigel," where I interview authors in front of an audience.

As we finished that evening I saw a familiar face looking at me from the crowd.

"Joe?" I said. It was one of my Dad's former producers. I hadn't seen him since my Dad's funeral.

"Hey, Jen!" he said. "It's so good to see you. I have to tell you I just loved your book, 'I'm Spiritual, Dammit!'"

Joe was a sports producer – not at all the type to be reading a humorous memoir about spirituality.

"It's so great to see you, Joe! How are things at the station?" I asked.

Joe hung his head.

"They let me go," he said. "It's been quite a struggle."

"No!" I said. I had no idea he was no longer a producer for CBS. "So where are you working now?"

Joe is a very talented guy. I had no doubt he'd been snatched up by another network.

"I've been doing a few things, actually," he said. "I do some writing and some broadcasting for the local high school, which doesn't pay much."

"So how are you making ends meet?" I asked.

"Well, I give out meat samples at Sam's Club on the weekends," he said.

Excuse me?!

"You're doing *what?*" I gasped, thinking he was kidding.

"It's not that bad, Jen," Joe continued, his voice getting a bit higher in pitch as if he were apologizing. "I mean, I get to meet so many wonderful people. And every shift is different. No job is beneath me being able to feed my family."

His last sentence lingered in the air like a mist.

"No job is beneath me being able to feed my family ..."

I felt like such an asshole. Here I was turning down a job to be on a major radio station doing traffic because I had done that job in '97, and this fabulous producer was giving out samples of processed meat at Sam's Club.

"You are an inspiration, Joe," I said. "You have no idea how much I needed to hear this."

On my way home, I called my agent.

"Put my hat in the ring for the traffic gig," I said.

No job is beneath being able to feed my family.

For some reason the only job on the table was this traffic position, and while my ego was saying, "You're above that, Jen!" perhaps the universe had a better plan. Maybe I was supposed to meet someone at that station who would change my life. Perhaps it would lead me to something even better. I had no idea, but I decided to get out of my own way and be the wide open field.

The one major issue with taking the traffic job was how I would figure out my childcare situation. Britt had just turned 5 and I was getting divorced. How would I get him to school if I was leaving for work at 3 a.m.?

Maybe my mom could move in?

While the thought of my mother moving into my tiny house wasn't my first choice, it was just about the only solution I could think of that made financial sense.

Maybe I'm not supposed to get divorced?

I wondered if this was God's way of telling me not to end my marriage.

Show me the next steps for my highest good and the highest good of all involved. No matter what it looks like, help me trust the signs and signals you send my way and help me let go of trying to control the process.

This had become my daily mantra. "Trusting the signs" was the hardest part for me to grasp, especially when the signs seem to suck.

Two days after I'd let my agent know about my accepting the traffic position, I got a call from a friend who worked for a media company.

"We're looking for a broadcast professional with writing experience for a new section we're launching," she said. "A lot of the writers we've interviewed have no broadcasting experience and a lot of the broadcasters can't write. You do both well, so we'd like to have you come in for an interview. What are you up to these days?" she asked.

"Well, it's funny you should ask, but I was just about to accept another position," I said.

"Can you come down for a chat before giving them an answer?"

Sure thing!!!

Accepting uncertainty or chaos, even when the situation seems really dire, can be extremely difficult. Think of the energy behind *acceptance:* it has a sort of neutral feeling, right? Whereas *giving up* because you're exhausted and have no other choice is sort of like screaming "FINE!!" while flipping off the sky. There's anger involved. You're clenching your fists and probably pissed at the world.

When you are in a neutral space, you're able to be the wide open field.

I once met a woman who compared *acceptance* to floating in the water with the tide instead of fighting against the waves.

"You can let the water carry you to safety, or you can fight until you're exhausted and then you drown," she said.

I went down for the meeting and wound up getting hired the next day.

"I can't believe the timing!" My mom said. "You're very lucky."

No, I just put my ego aside and got out of my own way.

❧ ❧ ❧

CHAPTER THREE
LOVE YOUR SHADOW

Facebook Status: "It's not your job to like me, it's mine."
– Byron Katie.

⚜ ⚜ ⚜

I don't think there is anything more depressing than winter in Chicago between January and March.

On one particular Friday it was not only snowy and blah, but the temperature was hovering around seven degrees. I was driving on a rather busy street on my way to work waiting at a red light, and I noticed a shivering woman standing at the bus stop holding a baby. They both looked like the wind chill was not only hurting their faces, but evaporating their souls.

What can I do to help?

I unrolled my window and shouted, "I know this may sound strange, but do you want a ride? I swear I'm not crazy, but you look so cold."

At first, the woman looked startled, and then her expression softened when she saw my smile. I could tell she was genuinely considering my gesture, until she looked in my backseat.

"You ain't got no baby seat," she said.

She was right – my son was too old for the booster chair that now sat in my garage.

I tried to think of a way to kidnap this frozen mother/daughter duo as the light turned green. Cars behind me leaned on their horns but I continued my conversation.

"I just don't want you guys to freeze," I said, thinking that in a different era, she'd not only hop into my car without a baby seat, but the child would probably be propped up on the hump in the middle to get the best view.

"Thanks anyways," she said, holding her child closer for warmth.

I pulled away and couldn't get the woman's face out of my mind. Was she a single mom? Did she have to take the bus to drop her child at daycare and then hop another bus to get to work? With all the struggles I was going through – ending my marriage and moving into a tiny little house – I couldn't imagine clutching my child for dear life at the bus stop in seven-degree weather.

"Our problems are "princess problems," my friend Jan often reminds me. "A REAL problem is not having a roof over your head or no job to go to."

A healer once told me we all have a team of angels just waiting to serve, but they have to be asked. I try to picture my angel team looking like the Commodores – a row of guys in classy white suits, moving in synchronized dance moves.

Hey angels, please send that woman and her child some of her own angels today. Help her feel warm and taken care of.

As I got to the highway, I was stopped dead in a traffic jam. I looked at the clock and it was after 9:30 a.m.

What the hell?

I turned on the radio to listen to the traffic report. The reporter made his way through the different tie-ups, and then said, "No delays on Lake Shore Drive ..."

No delays? What is he smoking?

I picked up my phone and dialed the traffic hotline. The one real perk from working as a traffic reporter for so long is I still had the number for the "Bat Phone." After two rings, one of my former colleagues picked it up.

"I'm sitting here not moving on Lake Shore Drive, and you just said 'no delays,'" I said. "What's up?"

"Oh come on, Jen, it's after 9:30; you know we don't give a shit," he joked. "Wait, an accident just came up on the screen," he said with a "this just in" urgency. "Looks like it's at Belmont in the left lane."

I was going to be late for work.

Princess problems.

I decided to spend my time sitting in traffic listening to my messages through the headset of my phone.

"Hey Jen, it's Gail. We're going to have to cancel the event we'd scheduled for you because the ticket sales have been kind of slow," she said.

I was scheduled to do a book talk/workshop at a community center in the suburbs the following week. I did these all the time; and while I can admit not every gig is standing room only, I've never had one cancelled because they can't sell tickets.

I'm such a loser.

Even though the spiritual side of me knows the mantras – *Don't take it personally. It's not about you. What you resist, persists,* (blah blah blah) the news that nobody wanted to come see me speak made this gloomy day even worse.

"It's a tough time of year to fill seats when it's this cold," Gail's message continued. "We'll plan something with you in the spring."

The traffic started to open up as a red Mercedes convertible cut me off. He had vanity plates touting his status as a CPA. The last time I saw a Mercedes with a vanity plate, it read: WIFELESS. (Did he think that was going to get him a date?)

DICKLESS would've been more appropriate.

I'm always fascinated by vanity plates. They're just so ... vain. Only once have I seen a vanity plate that made me smile. It was on a mini-van. The plate read BAGEL. It was driven by a sweet looking, elderly man who apparently loved his carbs.

I deleted Gail's message and went on to the next voicemail. It was from my lawyer.

"Hey Jen, it's Kristin. We have your court date. You'll be going in front of the judge on April 28th at 9 a.m. I'll email you the details but call me if you have any questions."

While my husband and I had been going through the process of divorce rather quickly (and amicably for the most part) hearing that there was an "end date" hit me hard.

As I clutched the steering wheel I started to feel my heart racing. My palms were sweating and I couldn't catch my breath.

What's wrong with me?

I suddenly felt nauseous and did my best to cut across three lanes of traffic so I could pull over. I put the car in park, and before I knew it tears started streaming down my face as I struggled to breathe.

I'm getting divorced.

For what felt like an eternity, I bawled my eyes out on the side of the road as my heart raced. Ten minutes went by before I felt confident that I could drive my car without veering off the road.

I called my therapist as soon as I got to work and told her what happened.

"You seem to have had a panic attack," she said. "How do you feel now?"

"OK," I said. "My heart rate is back to normal at least."

We made an appointment to chat the following morning and I went on with my day in a haze.

That night after work, I decided to stay home and watch a movie ... by myself.

Another Friday night, solo.

A friend had dropped off a bottle of champagne for me to "celebrate" my impending divorce, but I was in no mood for celebrating.

Should I have a glass of wine?

I'd spent a couple of years doing video production in the Napa Valley, so for a while, I was kind of a wine snob. When I got separated,

I started to use wine as a way to soothe stress or fall asleep. But I broke up with wine after I had my "ah-ha" moment:

One night when Britt was with his dad, I decided to open my best bottle of Cabernet. Somehow, I hoped a glass of $150 dollar wine would take my mind off of the fact that I was now living in a shoebox instead of the house of my dreams. Rather than have one or two glasses, I polished off the whole bottle. When the phone rang and I had trouble forming words, I was scared. I literally felt like I was floating above the scene, watching "drunk Jenny" try to be "smart, funny Jenny." I failed miserably, and told my friend I'd taken an Ambien. I then sat on the couch and got mad at myself.

What is wrong with you, Jen? You know better than this!

When I went to brush my teeth, my inner-monologue of self-judgment kept going.

You are so dumb to do this to yourself. How could you let this happen?

And then as I leaned down to spit out my toothpaste, I heard: "Love yourself. Don't leave yourself."

Oh God, now I'm hearing things? I knew I shouldn't have finished that bottle of wine.

"Love yourself. Don't leave yourself," that voice said again. It was loud and clear. And it stopped me cold in my tracks.

How can I love myself when I do something like this?

Human beings spend a lot of energy saving the whales and feeding starving kids, but when it comes to loving ourselves, we fail miserably.

I tried to imagine Britt as an adult. What if he felt so alone that he needed to choose to drink rather than love himself? Just the thought of this literally put tears in my eyes.

There's a book called "The Tools" written by two therapists: Barry Michels and Phil Stutz. They talk about loving your "shadow", which is all the stuff you don't want anyone to know about you. Whether it's how you behaved on prom night, or how you cheated on your wife, Stutz and Michels encourage everyone to stand side-by-side with that shadow and imagine him or her as your ally. We may have more than one shadow, too. Even if we have an entire "shadow team", we need to embrace them and picture them next to us, not hide them in a closet, deep down in our subconscious. When we include and love *all* the pieces of ourselves, we can finally be whole.

I remember when I told this theory to a friend of mine. She looked at me and frowned.

"I don't like my shadow," she said. "My shadow is a scared, abandoned, 7-year-old girl that wasn't loved or wanted. I don't want to bring her with me anywhere. I want to forget about her."

"If you were driving by a playground and saw a 7-year-old girl crying because she fell or was bullied, would you stop?" I asked.

"Of course," she said.

"But you won't accept that 7-year-old version of yourself who was neglected and unloved?" I said, "You are leaving her on the playground as she cries. You are abandoning the part of you that needs the most nurturing. 'The Tools' guys are saying we have to be there to nurture the part of ourselves that we're most ashamed of."

Sometimes our shame or fears run so deep, the thought of standing side-by-side with that shadow seems impossible.

So back to my solo Friday night: I was not following "The Tools" advice and was still beating myself up about a night from my past that I'd now named "The Cabernet Incident."

How could you have been so stupid!

I made myself some tea and decided that instead of ordering a movie, I should look through old photo albums.

This was probably not the smartest choice.

I woke at 2 a.m. on the couch, my wedding album in my lap and a box of Kleenex under my arm.

Later that morning, my mother stopped in for a visit.

"You look terrible," she said.

"I didn't get much sleep," I admitted.

We sat down with our coffee as I filled her in on everything, from my panic attack on Lake Shore Drive to my new court date.

"You could have crashed trying to drive during a panic attack," she said.

"I didn't plan to be driving, Mom. I've never *had* a panic attack before."

The conversation shifted to my impending court date, and as soon as I brought it up, my eyes started to water.

"Why are you crying? You filed for this divorce," my Mom said.

Just because someone files for divorce doesn't mean they wanted to get divorced.

"It's still sad, OK? I'm allowed to be sad at the ending of a 15-year relationship."

At this point, I could tell my mother was really uncomfortable with my crying. As a parent, I know how awful it is to see your kid sad. You want to make it stop at all costs. So here I was, my mother's child in tears, and she wanted to make things better.

"Honey, I think you need to seriously consider an antidepressant," she said, her voice getting stern.

I knew this was coming.

"I'm grieving a loss. This is healthy crying, alright?"

"I KNEW you would say that," my Mom said, her tone getting louder. "You are in denial. You are acting like CHARLIE SHEEN!"

"I'm what?!" I gasped.

Charlie Sheen? The guy who smokes "seven gram rocks" and lives with whores?

"How on earth am I acting like Charlie Sheen?"

"He won't take any medication, and he says he doesn't have a problem," she continued. "You are in denial just like he is."

I tried not to laugh.

"Mom, I appreciate your concern, but I am not in denial."

"Jen, I worry because you come from a long line of depressives," she said. "Your grandmother, my mother. And that's only on my mother's side! Who knows what the story was with my father and his clan?"

(My mother's father left town the day she was born, and managed to father 15 more children with about 14 different women throughout his brief lifetime. But that's a totally different book.)

"I have battled depression since my 20's," she continued. "It's a medical condition. Antidepressants have worked for me. It is not a drug that makes you loopy or eternally happy. You can be sad and cry ... you feel your pain ... It changes my perspective from a glass nearly empty to one that is half full."

"Mom, I get out of bed everyday, I go to work, get my kid to school, come home, make us dinner, and then go to bed. I'm functioning pretty well here. If I were a puddle on the floor not able to get out of the house for months, then you might have a point. But I already have a therapist. If she thought I needed to be medicated, it would have come up."

I understand that some people have medical conditions that require anti-depressants. I also think that as a society, we are choosing to pop way too many pills.

"Grief is healthy," I said, pointing to my tears. "I need to feel and I need to cry. Otherwise seven years later, I'll be walking down the bread aisle at the grocery store and snap for no apparent reason."

"What happened to Jen?"

"Oh, she took a bunch of Xanax during her divorce and couldn't feel her feelings. Delayed reaction."

I once wrote a story on anxiety, and Mark Pfeffer of the Panic/ Anxiety Recovery Center in Chicago told me, "You are allowed to be in a funk when you go through a loss or have something tragic happen to you. It's totally normal. But that should only last a few weeks. After that you have to pick yourself up from the bathroom floor and say, 'Enough!' And if you don't do this, your friends or family have a right to do it for you."

"Just promise me you won't rule it out," my mom insisted.

"I'm on it, Mom. I've been on top of this since the beginning with all the work I'm doing on myself."

My "pity-party" was almost over. And I was not lying on the bathroom floor.

But I did decide to cut my hair off.

"Will it come **back**?!" Britt gasped when I came home from the salon. "Where did it go?"

My hair hadn't been this short since the 8th grade, but there was something symbolic about getting all that dead hair off my shoulders.

⚜   ⚜   ⚜

On my court date a few weeks later, it was cold and dismal, just like my mood.

"Look your best, and hold your head high," my mom said. "Unfortunately, I have some experience in this department."

Entering the building where my proceedings were taking place, it seemed so sterile and impersonal. When I finally found my destination, I walked in and felt like I was in a bad episode of Judge Judy. Lawyers in cheap-looking suits filled the benches, along with really pissed off soon-to-be-ex-spouses.

My soon-to-be-ex and I sat together. We small-talked about Britt and the weather. I looked across the room and saw our lawyers in a huddle. There were only two female lawyers in the bunch and they were ours. After a few minutes, his lawyer approached us. She leaned into him to tell him something, her pleated pants two inches from my knee.

"She's claiming that there is only this much money in this account," she said, pointing to the numbers on the paper with her back in my face.

I can hear you, Bitch.

"That's fine," he said.

She walked away to go back and discuss some more details with my lawyer.

I looked around to see if any of the other couples were sitting together.

Nope.

This was a room full of broken dreams and broken hearts. Some people wiped away tears. Others looked enraged. The silence was deafening.

And our judge was late.

An hour after our designated time, she finally entered the court-room and asked us to approach the bench. We were shocked by her appearance. Her hair was so messy it looked like she'd stuck her hand in a light socket.

Is it that windy outside?

As we stood in front of our crazy-haired judge, things suddenly got surreal. She asked me a succession of quick-fire questions as she flipped through our file.

"Did you, Jenniffer Weigel, marry this man, on June 20th, 1998?" she barked, not looking up from her papers.

"Yes," I said.

My mind quickly flashed back to that hot summer day. I was so full of hope.

I still have my wedding dress in a "keepsake" box.

From the day our son was born to the moment I filed for divorce, every question she asked created a mini-movie in my mind.

"Yes, your honor," I kept saying in answer to her questions.

Is this really happening?

Fifteen years of laughs, birthdays, vacations, funerals and disagreements were now being summed up by a total stranger with bed-head.

And then, before I had a chance to catch my breath, she said,

"By the state of Illinois, this marriage is now dissolved ..."

Bang!

Her gavel hit the desk on "dissolved." I heard her voice echoing in my head long after she had finished speaking.

Dissolved?

The life I shared with my husband had been "dissolved" by the state of Illinois in four and a half minutes.

I turned to my lawyer to look for guidance.

Now what?

"I'll email you the final documents," my lawyers said.

"So that's it?" I asked.

"That's it," she said.

In a confused state I walked to the bench to get my coat and put it on. I threw my purse over my shoulder and made a beeline for the exit. Just before I made it to the door, I heard,

"Jenny!"

Jenny?

Only childhood friends, my family and my husband call me Jenny.

You aren't my husband anymore ...

He was standing there, holding his coat. He looked shell shocked. He reached to grab my arm. I could see tears in his eyes as he pulled me in for a hug.

Don't cry, Jen.

As we held each other I could hear him crying in my ear.

"Thanks," I said, trying to break the silence. "I really needed a hug today."

"Me too," he said, sniffing.

When we broke apart, I had trouble looking him in the eye.

"Bye," I said, feeling totally awkward and speechless.

"Yeah," he said.

I walked to the parking garage wondering what hit me. A slight drizzle of rain started to fall but I didn't have an umbrella. I let the wetness coat my hair and face, hoping it would help me feel my life. It didn't. Now I was cold *and* numb.

I got to work and tried to pretend it was just another day. Coming off the elevator, I passed by two female colleagues.

"Hey Jen," one of them said.

"Hey," I said, still in a haze.

"We're just bitching about our husbands," the other one said rolling her eyes.

I stopped walking, turned to them and said.

"I just got divorced."

There was an awkward pause, and then, "Oh my God, I'm *so* sorry," one of them said.

I tried to muster up a smile and kept walking until I reached my desk. There were a few texts from friends asking how it went. I called my mom and let her know I was OK.

"Go to dinner with friends, honey," she said. "Treat yourself."

But I was too sad to go anywhere but home.

That night, I saw an email from a friend trying to cheer me up.

"You have to watch this talk on TED," she wrote.

TED.com is where you can spend hours and hours watching authors, experts, scientists or humorists share their wisdom. The talk my friend sent me was called "The Power of Vulnerability" by author and therapist Brene Brown.

I clicked on the link and was quickly enthralled. In it, Brown discussed how she spent six years researching the topic of vulnerability through interviews, stories and focus groups.

"There was only one variable that separated the people who had a strong sense of love and belonging and the people who struggled for it; and that was, the people who have a strong sense of love and belonging believe they're *worthy* of love and belonging. That's it. They believe they're worthy," she said.

They're worthy..

She also looked at themes and patterns in that data. Those who had the strong sense of love and belonging also had a sense of courage.

"These folks had the courage to be imperfect," she said. "They had the compassion to be kind to themselves *first* and then to others, because you can't treat others kindly until you're kind to yourselves, and last they had a connection as a result of authenticity. They were willing to let go of who they *thought* they should be to be who they *were*. They fully embraced vulnerability. They believed that what made them vulnerable made them beautiful. They didn't talk about vulnerability being comfortable or excruciating – they just talked about it being necessary."

What made them vulnerable made them beautiful.

I was starting to see a theme. Being imperfect isn't wrong.

It's beautiful.

I'm imperfect, and I'm beautiful, dammit!

Chapter Four
Back in the Saddle

Heard on Michigan Avenue: "I don't even want to have lunch with the guy, let alone be handcuffed to his balcony!"

❧   ❧   ❧

You know you need to get laid when you start thinking about having "make-up sex" with your ex-husband.

"You should get back out there, Jen," my friends kept telling me. "Why not give online dating a shot?"

I know it's totally wrong, but I have this preconceived notion that only losers and people who have dead bodies stuffed in their trunks use online dating sites.

"What about a friend with benefits?" Another suggested.

I have a couple of friends who are really great guys. They are single and attractive but I wouldn't date them. Ever.

"Why not go to dinner with me?" One of them asked.

"I know too much," I said, remembering the story he told me about the threesome he had with a woman and her best friend on a recent trip to Vegas.

❧ ❧ ❧

One day I met my friend Bela Gandhi for lunch. Bela is the founder of "The Smart Dating Academy" who insists online dating would be my answer to long-term happiness.

"I have so many clients who are in super serious relationships that they found online," said Bela.

But I'm a full-time mom with a full-time job. I wasn't looking for something super serious.

"Some adult conversation and a movie that didn't feature Curious George – that's about all I can handle," I said.

"You can start up for a free trial," she said. "It's free. What do you have to lose?"

She kind of has a point.

Filling out the profile wasn't difficult until I got to the part where I had to describe myself. I write for a living and I couldn't for the life of me think of what to say. After several failed attempts I decided to ask Britt to write it for me.

"Honey, can you tell me all your favorite things about Mommy?" I asked.

He was drawing trucks with his crayons.

"I like when you make me mac and cheese," he said. "And I like when you sing me to sleep and how you read me books before bedtime. And I like you in dresses and not your jammies."

"Anything else?" I asked.

He shook his head, "no" and kept coloring.

Done.

I typed out Britt's answers and wrote them in my profile: "I was having a hard time writing about myself, so I asked my five-year-old to do it, and here's what he said …"

I thought it was hilarious. But judging by the freaks who responded immediately, I'm guessing a sense of humor doesn't translate well onto an online profile.

"People are going to think you're some weirdo who won't be able to exist without being attached at the hip to your kid," Bela said when I told her what I'd done. "You're a great mom. But you need to *show*, don't *tell*."

"What does that mean?" I asked.

"It means, tell a story about how you're dedicated to your son, and don't just say, 'I love my son.' Share an experience of you being adventurous; and don't just say, 'I'm adventurous.' Describe a time when you were loyal, rather than writing, 'my friends say I'm loyal.'"

After some tweaking, I was ready to go; so I launched the profile (penned by me and not my son.)

"What is your headline?" Bela asked me.

"My what?"

"You have to have a headline that grabs people," she said. "It's the one line that will be listed under your picture, so it should be short and sweet."

This is way too much work.

I went on the site to see what other people were using as headlines and couldn't believe my eyes.

"I want you to have my baby," said one.

"Your mother warned you about people like me!" said another.

"I'm bringing sexy back..." wrote a third.

What have I gotten myself into?

I decided to go with, "I believe in treating others the way I'd like to be treated."

"Good!" said Bela.

Within three minutes of completing the profile, I was inundated with emails. Nothing eloquent, mind you. Phrases like, "Hey cutie!" or "What-up?" were commonplace. One man even said "Send me some body pics, babe! Wanna see if your (sic) hot from the waist down too."

What?!

"One in twenty emails will be worth your while," stressed Bela. "That means you'll have to weed through dozens of bad ones to find the good. Be patient."

As the days went on, more emails came through. Several men had photos of themselves wearing no shirts while sitting at their computer.

Seriously?

(Note to men everywhere: It's never ever OK to take pictures of yourself partially clothed for your online dating profile – especially if you're sitting in a chair at your computer. If you want to show off your six-pack-abs, be DOING something, like swimming or fishing or rock climbing. Even then, you come off as arrogant, but at least you are taking part in an activity and not just posing. But a man sitting at his desk chair with no shirt just brings out all sorts of bad images that you don't want anyone to have in a first impression.)

After weeding through the partially clothed pictures, I found more shocking headlines.

"I need a wife now."

Delete.

"This must be your lucky day."

Delete

"I'm back in the saddle after 40 years of marriage and ready for action."

Delete.

Bad jokes were abundant. Typos eventually became something I'd expect with every transaction. Also, the only men who reached out to me were either way too old or way too young. My peers seemed to only want women in their 20's. I was pretty popular with young dudes looking for cougars and the old men (we're talking ages 65-89) looking for someone who would make them want to pop a Viagra.

But then, one email came peeking through that seemed promising. He didn't write words like "pornography" or "coolio" in the first paragraph. And he was my age. I shot him a note that maybe coffee could be in our future.

As I waited for a response, I admit, I started getting a little excited. The last time I dated I was driving a stick shift and checking for messages on my answering machine from a pay phone. While the concept of small talk with a stranger sounded exhausting, something about this man seemed genuine. Perhaps if anything, I'd make a new friend out of the deal?

Soon, I found a reply in my in-box.

"I'm looking to meet a woman who has been divorced for a couple of years, so we're just not the right fit for each other right now. Best wishes to you."

Best wishes??!! OMG- my first online dating rejection and he doesn't even know my real name!

I was so pissed, I was about to give up completely. After taking a couple of days to cool off I went back to my in-box to see if anything caught my interest.

And there he was.

He expressed an interest in things I mentioned in my profile. He used correct grammar. He commented on the look on my face in one of my photos. And he was my age.

I looked him up. He was handsome, but not stunning. Tall, which I love. He'd been divorced two and a half years, had two kids under the age of 10, and most importantly, he was employed. Not just any job either. He ran a large company in Chicago.

"Don't screw it up," my Mom said when I told her I was meeting him for dinner.

The day of our first date I was a nervous wreck. When I arrived I saw a single man with brown hair sitting alone.

"Are you Dan?" I asked.

"Nein" He said in a heavy German accent. (Which I'm guessing means "no")

At that moment, a man in a navy blue suit came from around the corner to introduce himself.

"I'm Dan," he said, reaching out to shake my hand. He was very attractive in person. (And did I mention his suit? There's something about a man in a perfectly tailored suit ...) "I bet that guy is kicking himself right now," he added, looking at the confused German man I'd left behind.

Conversation was effortless. We even chose the same items on the menu. I started wondering why I hadn't tried getting out into the dating scene sooner,

As he walked me to my car we passed by a homeless man. He reached in his pocket and pulled out a 20 dollar bill.

"I'm not trying to impress you or anything," he said.

Yeah, right.

"I sort of have a problem where I always do this," he said, handing the man his money.

The homeless guy looked down, expecting a single or maybe a five, but was blown away by the amount now in his hand.

"Oh bless you, man!" He gushed. The homeless man then looked at me and said, "You've got yourself a good man!"

As soon as he said this, I got a horrible feeling in the pit of my stomach. While at first I tried to chalk it up to the calamari we'd shared at the restaurant, I quickly realized it wasn't a bad food pain, but my internal "look out" radar detector. I've had a sensitive stomach since I came out of the womb. My "gut check" as I call it has gotten me out of many tricky situations or bad relationships. Learning to trust that gut has served me well. But this date had been too awesome for me to accept it in this circumstance.

Maybe my gut is wrong?

He kissed me on the cheek as we parted, and as I was on my way home, there was already a message waiting on my blackberry.

"Is it too soon to ask when I can see you again?" He wrote.

Dating is fun!

For the next few weeks, he showered me with emails and text messages. If he had thirty minutes between clients, we would meet for coffee by my office.

"Are you going to introduce him to Britt?" My friends would ask.

Meeting people my parents were dating when I was a kid was an unsettling process. It's not that my parents dated awful people, but they would use my brother and me to gauge whether or not the girlfriend/boyfriend was a keeper. If they liked kids, they would last longer. If they were annoyed by a trip to the Lincoln Park Zoo, they were gonners.

If I were "King of the World" I would make it illegal to drag your kids along while you try to find a life partner. If someone treats you well and makes you happy, chances are they will treat your children well and make them happy too. Bringing the kids in the mix too soon is just harder for everyone, and completely irresponsible.

Both my ex and I made an agreement that we weren't going to introduce Britt to anyone we were seeing unless we were absolutely serious about them. My ex had been dating but he assured me there would be no introductions to Britt.

I sent him an email saying I was considering allowing Britt to meet Dan's kids at a park in a very neutral "this is my friend Dan and his two kids" kind of environment. Not as my boyfriend, mind you. Just as a male friend.

He responded with "I'm still not comfortable talking to each other about our dating life, but I trust your judgment as I hope you would trust mine."

Meanwhile, back to my life with Dan, I soon found myself becoming a text-message addict. I would anxiously wait to hear from my new friend and he would do the same. It was totally intoxicating.

"Remember that the oxytocin that pumps through your body in the early stages of dating is like a drug, so whatever you do, don't give in and have sex too soon," Bela told me. "You have to make sure the emotional connection is mutual before you make a physical connection."

We had such a hard time aligning our schedules anyhow. But I had to admit, in the back of my mind, I was hopeful our timing would eventually allow for some physical contact.

"How soon is too soon?" I asked. "My waxing lady is really hard to get into; I need to plan ahead," I joked.

"Well, men take a lot longer to get emotionally connected than women, so to be really safe, I recommend that people wait at least 12 dates," she said.

12 DATES?!

"Yes. The clients who have had long-term success with a match don't give it up until the 12th date."

I was really starved for sex, so this sounded like an impossible task. But even more alarming than the 12-date rule was the fact that my "gut check" wouldn't stop giving me warning signs about this guy. I'd try to convince myself that the ache in my stomach was just in my head. Dan seemed like such a great guy on the surface (and he looked so good in those suits). It's not like I thought he was a serial killer, I just had a feeling he was hiding something.

Whatever Jen. You're just out of practice!

I continued to ignore my internal security system and stayed in touch with my new friend. And then out of nowhere, I noticed a complete 180-degree change in his behavior. He went from texting me several times a day to total silence.

Since I hadn't dated in this digital age, I went to a younger colleague and asked her for advice. I showed her my phone so she could read all transactions and give me her honest opinion.

"Something is definitely up," she said, literally targeting the text where his attitude went from "excited to chat" to "I couldn't care less." "You didn't change a thing and he totally switched tone. He's playing games."

I'm too old for this shit.

I filled Bela in on the correspondence and she suggested I meet him in person before making assumptions.

"The emotional rollercoaster becomes more severe when we text," she said. "Ninety-three percent of how we interpret people is through the non-verbal exchange – the tone of their voice, facial expression, posture. Only seven percent is through words; so when you're texting, you only have that seven percent to work with. Meet him face-to-face and then you'll know for sure."

I tried to arrange a coffee date, but he wouldn't commit to any face-to-face time. He blamed it on work and his busy schedule.

"He was making time for you when he was slammed," my co-worker reminded me. "If someone wants to see you, they make time to see you. Period. He's full of it."

As I was driving in to work totally frustrated that I couldn't reach Dan, I felt like I was flashing back to high school.

"I'm a grown woman, and I'm taking this rejection as if I were a 16-year-old girl!" I told my friend Laura.

What the hell is going on here?

I started to pray on my way into work like I hadn't prayed in months.

Please universe. Help me heal this ache in my heart. Help me so I feel in control. I need to feel in control again. This is too painful. Give me the strength to feel OK. Let me know it's going to be OK. You are stronger than this, Jen. Be strong.

Within seconds of finishing my prayer, my friend John St. Augustine called.

"How's it going?" He asked.

I vented and he listened until it was time for me to park my car and go into work. When I arrived at my desk, there was already an email from him with words of wisdom.

"I heard this loud and clear after we hung up – so here it goes," he wrote. **"It's about you..It's about you...It's about you**. He is playing his role perfectly...as you are with him. Whether he knows it or not – it matters not. But the bottom line is this: It's too soon for you.... there's much healing and inner work that needs to take place for you. **Become complete without needing another**. Then the illusion of being abandoned will be gone. You are being forced to confront your greatest fear. The roots are deep. You are more conscious now than any of your family before you...That's why it hurts so much. You can't drink it away, screw it away, spend it away, or pray it away."

I can't pray it away? God dammit!

"You cannot be holy with another until you are whole with yourself. Sit down with that little Jenniffer that is inside, so full of hurt and pain and rage ... as her friend and partner ... listen to what she has to say ... and forgive the unforgivable."

Forgive the unforgivable.

I silently wondered how much hurt one person could take in a lifetime before choosing to drive their car into oncoming traffic. I knew that any rejection that I faced reminded me of the abandonment I felt as a child. When my Dad moved out. When my step dad moved out. It's a reminder of all the wounds caused by men disappointing me at different stages in my life.

Does the inner child ever get healed?

While I knew Dan wasn't the perfect man for me, after so many months of solitude, I felt like someone was better than no one.

Right?

And after watching my own life implode, it felt good to daydream about a new life with a new person. (Complete with a big house in the suburbs and a lake house in Michigan.)

All this after just a month of knowing someone.

Man, am I out of practice.

I finally nailed Dan down for a breakfast. He was cold and weird and could barely look me in the eye.

"Just tell me what's going on," I said. "If you don't want to spend time with me, I can handle it. But don't avoid me and make excuses."

He admitted that he ran into his ex on the train and it really threw him for a loop.

"Your ex-wife?" I asked.

"No, the woman I was seeing after my marriage ended," he said. "I've never loved anyone so much or tried to make something work so hard in my life, and it just didn't work out. That was so devastating. And seeing her made me realize I'm not totally over it."

His words lingered in the air like a cloud of exhaust... "I've never loved anyone so much or tried to make something work so hard in my life ..."

*You loved this woman and tried harder to make it work with her than you did with the mother of your two kids?? **What an asshole!***

When I got back to my desk after the confession chat, I kept alternating between feeling like I was going to throw up, to wanting to punch him in the nuts.

Why didn't I trust my gut?

Then as if on cue, there was an email from a friend of mine with the subject "Not good." See, when I was having trouble pinning Dan down for a person-to-person chat, I decided to send out emails to all the women I knew who lived in the area where he once lived with his wife. (I am a reporter, after all.) Turns out, one of my friends knew Dan's ex-wife. (What are the chances?) And while I know there are two sides to every story, Dan had a rap sheet a mile long. Several people referred to him as "cheater-cheater pumpkin eater" and explained he had mistresses far and wide, often taking them with him on business trips across the globe. That girlfriend he was referring to was the affair that broke up his marriage.

And you know what they say about cheaters …

I sure know how to pick em.

This man also had "the smallest penis on the planet" according to his ex-wife and a few other women he had dated, my friend wrote in the email.

Oh Jesus!

My gut may have been right, but it didn't make me feel any better.

The next day, I cancelled my online dating subscription.

⚜   ⚜   ⚜

A couple weeks after what I soon labeled "the online dating debacle," my friend insisted on setting me up with a guy she knew.

"He's not divorced yet, but separated," she said.

One thing I learned from the online dating world is "separated" often means "I think I want to leave my wife, but first I need to see what's out there and make sure I have someone better to jump into bed with."

"Tell him to call me when he's divorced," I said.

"Come on," she insisted. "His wife is dragging her heels but he's already moved out, and it's totally over between them."

Although I was still playing the "it's too soon" game, we arranged to meet at a restaurant for dinner.

I knew it wasn't going to end well when he insisted on cutting my meat.

"Do my arms look broken?" I asked, my jaw slightly dropping as he muscled his way through my filet.

"Just let somebody else take control for once," he said, as if I'd known him a lifetime instead of a mere 30 minutes.

I refused his proposal for an after dinner drink in his hot tub, so the date quickly came to an end.

"Seriously Jen, I have the perfect guy for you," said a co-worker.

If I had a nickel for every time I've heard that since my divorce ...

"What does he do?" I asked.

"He's in the military," she said. "He's forty-two, never been married, and very successful."

I actually think if you're over 40 and you've never been married, or at least really close to being married, you probably have some serious issues that I don't feel like taking on at this stage in my life.

"What's wrong with him?" I asked.

"Nothing," she said. "I swear ... I think you guys would get along great."

My stomach was a mess just thinking about this. The thought of another blind date made me want to blow chunks.

Rather than listening to my gut, however, I arranged to meet this man after work for dinner.

He was very stunning – showed up right on time, and was in full military attire.

"You shouldn't have gotten so dressed up for little ole' me," I joked.

He barely cracked a smile and claimed to have come straight from a graduation ceremony, which required that he be in uniform.

Then the skeptic in me stepped in. What if he is some unemployed dude who just stopped by a costume shop and rented the military garb? Anyone could rent a Navy Captain suit, right?

Why do you keep doing this??

Not only did this guy have zero sense of humor, but right out of the gate I noticed he was incredibly awkward and nervous – almost as if he'd never done this before. He described himself as tenacious.

"The only difference between me and a pit bull is, the pit bull will eventually let go."

Stalker, party of one, your table is ready!

As if the pit bull comment weren't bad enough, early into the meal after our conversation seemed to steer in the direction of moral beliefs and religious backgrounds for some crazy reason – (he is super-Catholic and I wrote a book called, "I'm Spiritual, Dammit!") – he drops this bomb:

"I'm a virgin."

Holy shit. I'm out with the REAL 42-year-old virgin.

Have you ever been in a situation where you would do anything – absolutely anything – to be able to push a button that would immediately remove you from your current location and land you on your couch with your snuggly blanket and a nice bowl of ice cream?

When he went to the bathroom, I texted my friend Jan to call me in five minutes so I could fake an emergency.

Five minutes later my phone vibrated, right on cue.

"I have an emergency and I need to leave," I lied. "I am SOOO sorry," I said as I grabbed my coat.

Something tells me I wasn't the first woman to do this to him, by the way.

Within hours, I put the memo out to my inner circle to stop setting me up with people. Period.

"You didn't give it enough time," said Bela. "If you joined a gym and didn't lose all the weight you wanted right away, would you quit your gym membership?"

Maybe

"You're too picky," my mom said after I filled her in on my encounters.

"Too picky?" I gasped. "You liked Dan and he wound up being a sociopath!"

"Everyone has flaws," she said.

"I'm not ready," I said. "If it's meant to be, I'll run into someone on the elevator or walking down the street."

"You have to keep trying," Bela insisted.

"No thanks," I said.

⚜ ⚜ ⚜

After the dust settled with my dating woes, I sent my ex an email.

"I just wanted you to know that Britt won't be meeting any male friends at this time," I wrote. "I figured I would want to know if the tables were turned."

He responded right away.

"I'm sorry things didn't work out with him. But I'm sure you'll find someone eventually who will make you happy."

I read into that email every way from Sunday. First, I thought it was sweet. Then I thought it was condescending and I added a lilt to his voice with the "SOMEONE" every time I read it.

I went back to my email from John St. Augustine.

Become complete without needing another. Then the illusion of being abandoned will be gone.

"The only someone who will fill that hole and make me feel whole is me," I wrote back in an email to my ex.

So the man I plan to date right now is Britt. And maybe Sponge Bob Square Pants ... (although he doesn't look quite as good in a suit).

⚜   ⚜   ⚜

CHAPTER FIVE
KICKED OUT OF HEAVEN

Facebook Status:

Heard on Michigan Avenue: "If I died, I would definitely come back and haunt the shit out of people."

"Why?"

"I'd be dead so I wouldn't have any other skills."

☙ ☙ ☙

"Hey Jen, wanna meet a woman who was kicked out of heaven?"

Huh?

I was reading my emails and a friend was inviting me to come to Evanston Hospital. An orthopedic surgeon was scheduled to speak in the hospital auditorium to tell her story of how she died in a kayaking accident and was "kicked out" of heaven. She had "work left to do on earth" or something.

While this sounded interesting, I had another important engagement.

"It's Britt's birthday," I wrote her back. My son's birthday trumped any weekend activity ... even a lady who said she died and came back to life.

Two days later I received an email from a PR person promoting the same talk at a hospital. While my work as a columnist meant getting dozens of pitches a day, I never received any emails from the "I See Dead People" crowd.

"Please consider Dr. Mary Neal for a story," the email read.

Maybe I'm supposed to meet this woman.

As I read on and learned more about her, I discovered that Mary was skeptical of near-death experiences, or NDE's as the folks who died and came back call them, until she was trapped underwater for nearly 30 minutes. While dead, she said she floated above the scene and saw her lifeless body. In her book *To Heaven and Back* she talks about her death from a doctor's point of view:

"(My death) was a relatively slow process during which I was conscious, alert and fully aware of what was happening. It sounds rather morbid, but from an orthopedic surgeon's perspective, I was intrigued as I felt my knee bones break and my ligaments tear. I tried to analyze the sensations and consider which structures were likely involved. I seemed to feel no pain but wondered if I was actually screaming without knowing it. I did a quick self-assessment and decided I was not screaming. I felt curiously blissful, which is remarkable because I had always been terrified of drowning."

Mary says she encountered a group of what she believed to be souls. She was taken "along a brilliant and beautiful path that led to a great dome-like structure that was, indeed, brilliant and exploding with the pure and complete love of God", but she wasn't allowed to stay. She was told she had things to take care of on earth.

Mary was now traveling the country sharing her story with anyone who would listen, especially the skeptics in the medical community.

She was coming through Chicago to be the keynote speaker at a hospital in Evanston for the monthly meeting of IANDS- International Association of Near Death Studies.

"Is there any chance Dr. Neal can come down to the city so I can meet her during my lunch hour?" I wrote to the PR agency. "I'd like to interview her for my book."

Within minutes I had a response that Mary would be joining me later that day.

"Wanna meet a doctor who died and came back to life?" I wrote to my co-worker, Pete, in an email.

Pete had read both of my books and was the only person at work I could talk to about my fascination with all things metaphysical and spiritual. Since I'd interviewed several people for my first two books who claimed they talked to the dead, I figured a real doctor could have some credibility.

"Absolutely!" Pete responded.

Mary greeted us in the lobby with the most beautiful smile, tanned skin and piercing blue eyes.

"So great to meet you!" She beamed.

I started to wonder if "seeing the light" had rubbed off on her somehow because she was glowing – in a big way. It almost felt like I needed to wear sunglasses.

We went to the cafeteria and found a table by the window. The television on the wall was up full volume as a woman on The Maury Povich Show charged at another woman. They both lost their hair weaves in the struggle.

"You betta BEEP BEEP BEEP you BEEEEEEEEPPPP!!!!"

I tried to ignore the women bitch-slapping each other to focus on my conversation. I then realized I was in the middle of two totally opposite worlds: The television show from hell and a lady who said she'd been to heaven.

Pete got us beverages and I took out my recording device.

"So Mary, after everything you've experienced, do you feel your perceptions of life are totally different?" I asked.

"Absolutely," she said. "There are many things that have changed. Very concretely I no longer fear death – my own death or the death of people I love. And I was reasonably tolerant beforehand, but since this happened I am entirely tolerant of people now. I know that God loves me unconditionally and loves everyone else unconditionally too."

I looked up at the television. The women were now hitting each other as Maury sat there smirking.

God really loves everyone. Even assholes on the Maury Povich Show?

"I am now able to be tolerant and forgiving toward people I don't even particularly like. And that's a very concrete change. You look at every minute of every day because every minute really matters – every choice we make, every action we take, they really matter. I feel that when we are here on earth, we have this incredible opportunity to learn and grow and help others on their path. Whether it's developing tolerance or love or compassion – or helping someone develop compassion – God has a purpose and plan for each one of us. It's a big deal to try to listen for those next steps and an even bigger deal to try to obey."

"Do you ever have moments where you don't want to listen?" I asked.

"Well of course," she said. "Coming and talking to you today – that was really 'obeying.' This is not my cup of tea. I mean, I am an orthopedic surgeon. I have a husband; I have kids; I have a very busy life. Writing a book is something I had no desire to do. I am not a writer. I didn't want to be a writer. I am a pragmatist, a concrete thinker; I'm not given to fanciful ideas. I am not creative. I couldn't dream up this story if I tried. But when I was kicked out of heaven ..."

"Kicked out?" I asked.

"Yes. I was told I had to "go back" because I had work to do," Mary said.

I thought abandonment from the men in my life was tough to handle. A rejection from heaven would send me into a full-blown crisis.

There aren't enough shrinks in the world ...

"I was given the task of sharing my story as a way of helping others find their way back to God," she explained. "But when I was dead and in the light, I had no desire to come back to this life. I love my husband and kids intensely. But I was not interested in coming back to this life."

"Based on what you've read – other near-death experiences – I'm wondering if you see yours as different?" Pete asked.

"No. I think mine is more extensive in its entirety than most people's, but again, I'm a rationalist, I'm a scientist, I read extensively. This happened in 1999. It has been 13 years, and in that period of time I have read and talked to many people. I see tons of patients every week, and I would say every week there are at least two patients who come in and say 'I heard you had an after-death experience; can I tell you what happened to me?' Almost every experience talks about the pervasiveness and intensity of love and this incredible beauty."

"There are many who think a near death experience is just oxygen missing from the brain," I said. "What do you say to that?"

"I was dead for far too long for this to be something that was caused by a lack of oxygen," Mary said. "And the presence of something more was far too vivid."

"So ... is it solely a Christian perspective for you?" Pete asked.

"Yes and no. It's difficult for me to answer that. I know that my job is to get my story out because I've seen the power it has to change peoples lives; but I also know that I've done a number of interviews, and there is a large part of the American population that is focused on dogma; and if you don't follow that dogma specifically they discount the entire experience."

I thought about Mary's words. For me, I was raised a Christian – but our faith depended on who my Dad was married to at the time. We started off Methodist when he was married to my mom; became Episcopalians with wife number two; we ended up Congregationalist with his third wife, which meant we just made appearances on Easter and Christmas Eve. It felt to me as though people were using the church as an excuse for being a jackass Monday through Saturday, so I stopped going.

"Were you raised a Christian?" Pete asked. Pete was raised a Southern Baptist and was admittedly still recovering.

"I was raised to go to church on Sundays," Mary said. "After the service we would stand on the front steps of the church for a few minutes, then go back to our lives. Religion was never discussed in my home. I was not a non-believer, but I wasn't consciously spiritual on a daily basis."

I found it refreshing that Mary was talking about having a brush with heaven, yet she wasn't "in-your- face" about religion. I tell my son that God can find you if you're sitting on the toilet ... and to treat others the way you'd like to be treated. Period. As for the holy scripture, I suspect that stories in the Bible have "evolved" over time. (How many editors do you suppose got their hands on the Good Book?) Case in point: my family can mess up a story after 20 minutes. It's like a bad game of "telephone". Whatever your beliefs, there is no doubt that Jesus was onto something. What really bothers me are all the people who claim to live by his teachings but who don't act very Jesusy. Another thing: Christ was forgiving. I have known of a lot of judgmental Christians. That **really** pisses me off.

"Am I a Christian? Yes," Mary continued. "Having said that, the frustration for me with Christianity is that so many people worship Christ and not God. Christ bridged the gap for us, but it all comes down to God. Christ tried to show us that God actually loves us. My experience doesn't fit entirely with Christian dogma. But I'm still an absolute believer in organized religion."

"But doesn't organized religion promote segregation?" I asked.

"I think there's a very important role for organized religion," Mary said. "I think the denominations are great because God meets you where you are, wherever that is. But where I think the denominations get stuck is when each one says 'we know the real deal; we know how to interpret the Bible and you don't.'"

"My sister was never baptized, yet she goes to a Catholic school," I said. "There are those who think she's going to hell because of that."

Mary shook her head. "If I grew up in India I'd be a Hindi, and if I grew up in Pakistan I'd probably be a Muslim. I think one of the problems is that humans are so limited in their thinking. We just don't get it. We can't understand how big God really is. The idea that a loving God is going to look at someone who grew up as a

Muslim and not love that person is not the reality. That is not consistent with anything that has historically been written about God."

"So you have skeptics among Christians AND among people in your field?" Pete asked.

Mary took a deep breath and smiled.

"Well, It's really interesting. When I did a book signing at a hospital recently, out of the 46 physicians on staff, only one showed up. But I know what I know, and if you look back at the history of medicine, it's only been in recent years that there's this schism between medicine and spirituality. In the old days the spiritual leader and the medical person were one in the same. I would say that medicine is beginning to come around now, in that medical schools are incorporating mind-body connections, but it's definitely on the fringes. The more people from scientific backgrounds who talk about the spiritual component in relation to medicine, the more acceptable it will become. As the push becomes more to wellness instead of fixing problems when they arise, the spiritual component by necessity will be more prevalent. I see this in my own practice. I address patients' spiritual needs more than I did in the past and my patients do better. I also was blessed to have had some spiritual experiences throughout my life *before* the near-death experience."

"What kind of spiritual experiences?" I asked.

"When my son was four or five, I said something about what he would do when he was 18 and he said, 'I'm never going to make it to 18, mom.' I asked him, 'What do you mean?' He looked at me with confusion, **like, 'Don't you know? That's part of the plan.'** He couldn't believe that I didn't know that. I think young kids have a very different connection to God's world. One of the reasons given to me on why I was to return to earth after my accident was that it was my responsibility to be this spiritual rock for everyone else during my son's death, because I was told that my son would die young."

Mary not only had the difficult journey of trying to heal from her severe injuries; she was told by spirits who took her down the path that she would need to help her family with the passing of her son.

"How many years was it that you had this knowledge your son was going to die?" I asked.

"About 10 years," Mary said.

My eyes welled up.

"And how was the anticipation leading up to your son's 18th birthday?" I asked.

"Oh it was horrible! The summer before, there was another boy in our community who had this car accident. He was hit, head-on, and he died. I didn't know the boy; but the night he died I had a dream where this same boy came to me and said he traded places with my son. He said his work was done, but that my son's was not. I woke up thinking, 'That's weird.' That morning, I see the kid's picture in the paper with the story of how he had died. I knew then that he was the boy in my dream. Eventually, my son's 18th birthday came and went, and he was still alive. But I cherished every minute of every day with him."

"But he still died young?" I asked.

"He passed at 19, yes," she said.

"So you got a year longer with him than you thought you would; but that's still so devastating. How did your husband handle all this?"

"I didn't tell my husband until about six months before my son's 18th birthday, because I didn't want him to think about it. "When I finally did, he wasn't happy.""

No kidding.

"But the morning of my son's 18th birthday, we were in West Yellowstone, and I went over to my son's hotel room at four a.m. just to wake him up and see that he was still with us. Then I actually told him the whole story about what he'd told me as a child, about not making it to 18, and the other boy who told me in my dream he'd traded places with my son."

I looked at the table next to us, which was full of people, and wondered if they were hearing any of our conversation. I started to worry that maybe they thought we'd all lost our minds, until I realized they were glued to Maury.

"Why do you think that other boy traded places with him?" I asked.

Mary sighed and held up her hand, expanding her fingers.

"What I was shown when I died was that we have these branch points where we can exit our life, and my son hit this branch point, and his work wasn't done. The other boy's was. So he traded places with my son, which gave him an extra year and a half. In the few days leading up to my son's death he had all these conversations with people about what they think happens when we die. Nineteen-year-old kids don't do that. He asked me about a Will and life insurance. And on the day he died, he was roller-skiing with a friend and they passed a cemetery. He told her the story of him saying he wasn't going to live to be 18. He then gave her very specific instructions as to what he wanted done, were he to die. They roller-skied a bit further, and then they stopped at this overlook to admire the beautiful day. Just before they took off again he said, 'Wouldn't this be great to be the last thing you ever saw?' A minute later he was dead."

Pete and I sat there in stunned silence. Here was a woman of science talking about branch points and messages from dreams.

Crazy – party of one – your table's ready.

Yet somehow, I knew this doctor was far from nuts. She was absolutely certain that what she was telling us was the truth. And after learning that she had to bury one of her children, I wondered how she could be so upbeat.

"Why do you think bad things happen to good people?" I asked.

"I don't believe there's such a thing as good and bad," she said.

What?

"Everyday I read about people who are killed in the news. How could this not be bad?" I asked.

"You get your BEEP BEEP BEEP ass over here you BEEP BEEP BEEP!!" a woman on the television yelled.

Maury was catering to idiots. Definitely bad.

"I can't tell you how many times over the last 13 years, where something terrible has happened, where someone says 'isn't that terrible about that boating accident?' and I think, 'No actually, it's a great gift.'"

"A tragedy is a great gift?" I wanted clarification.

"If you think about bad things, think about Jesus: he was betrayed, he was arrested, he was beaten, humiliated, and then he was killed.

80

That's bad! By all accounts we should look at that and say 'that's the most horrible thing you can imagine.' But look what came of it. For more than 2000 years people have passed along his story and his beliefs, using them to heal and love. How can you look at that and say it's horrible? I look at the affect Jesus has had, and it's incredible. He brought a covenant of love to this earth."

Watching my Dad die on Father's Day at the age of 56 was horrific. But it did send me on a spiritual journey that never would have taken place, otherwise.

"You can look at every bad thing that has happened and almost always there are incredibly good things that have come out of it," Mary said. "You know change doesn't happen when things are easy. Change happens when things aren't easy and when you are pushed. So I would say there is no such thing as good and bad. They just ... are. And we may not be able to make sense of it."

It's easy to tell people that there is no such thing as bad when you've been to heaven and back, but what about the rest of us stuck in this sludge we call life?

"Your experience has helped you see this," I said. "It's kind of hard for those going through the daily grind to see a murder or being stuck in traffic as not bad things."

"Maybe you're stuck in traffic because you are being saved from an accident miles down the road," Mary said. "People rarely think of the other side of an inconvenience; but even when we are in an uncomfortable situation there is a reason. Maybe you're being spared a much worse situation down the line, or you are supposed to meet someone at a certain time. I like to describe it this way: there's this huge, incredibly intricate tapestry that is beautiful. Imagine that you are one little thread. You can't see that you're part of this tapestry; you're just a thread. And an you're thinking, 'oh my gosh, I'm getting frayed over here.' We don't have the capacity to see the big picture. Not when we're in the thick of it."

"And that's when we don't bless our mess," I said.

"Yes, because we don't have the bird's eye view. If you think about being raised with faith when you're a little kid, you have hope. You hope that God will do what he says he will do. Then you go through life and that hope transforms into faith. And that's usually where most people stay. But if you have a profound experience like I did, then that faith transforms into an absolute trust. And that trust is really what changes your life. Because I *trust* that there is that beautiful tapestry. I don't even ask any more why something happens. I just go with it. I have that trust. Yeah. Ok. It is part of this overall beautiful tapestry, and someday I will see the tapestry."

"Do you trust, or do you know?" Pete asked.

"I know that there's a tapestry," she said. "I trust that what's happening at any moment in time is part of that tapestry. My brother-in-law just died; so I look at that and figure that 'I don't know what part his death plays, but I have absolute trust that it is part of the bigger scheme. I trust that it is part of something bigger."

"Is there anything in your experience that led you to refute or confirm the idea of reincarnation?" Pete asked.

"I didn't give it a whole lot of thought before this," Mary said. "I do think we have this incredible opportunity to come here. I do think that before you come into a life, there's this outline that is created, and it's like talking to your college advisor when you're trying to figure out your college courses. The family you come into is also very specific."

This reminded me of my conversation with "The Four Agreements" author, don Miguel Ruiz. He told me that we choose our parents. I still have a difficult time accepting that I chose a dad who would die from a brain tumor at a relatively young age. Perhaps Dad chose to "exit" when he did, because it would have been too difficult to beat brain cancer or live the life he would have wanted after his surgeries? Just trying to make sense of it.

I then wondered if Mary had heard of "The Four Agreements" or any of the spiritual books I'd read and enjoyed.

"What do you think of some of the so-called 'new age' teachings that are out there now?" I asked.

"I think that a lot of the new-age stuff is a mistake because it's all about 'me' and how 'I can become God.' I believe God is in all of us but that doesn't mean we can become God."

I started to think that maybe Mary would like Wayne Dyer's acronym about the ego: Edging God Out.

"I hate you, you dumb BEEP BEEP BEEP!! I swear if you even BEEP over BEEP I will BEEP you BEEP BEEP!" A lady was screaming hysterically on TV.

Hell was up full volume during my brush with heaven.

"So where are people on the other side?" I asked, quietly wishing the ladies hitting each other on Maury were anywhere but this side of the veil.

"I think there are angels all around us," Mary said. "I do think that people come in and out of your lives when they are supposed to, and that there is an overall plan. I don't believe in pre-destiny because there's something very powerful about free choice; but as I mentioned, we have these branch points where we can exit if we choose. I think the fear of death or the fear of another person's death can really limit our ability to live."

The fear of death limits our ability to live.

"Why do you think it's so hard for humans to accept your experience?" Pete asked. "Is it culture, or humans or... It's a rhetorical question really. But I do wonder."

"I think developed countries are less able and less willing to think about spiritual issues," Mary said. "I mean, we can embrace radio waves. We can't see them but we believe they exist. But we can't accept a near death experience? I think life becomes too busy. There's too much static on the line. The more simple your life, the easier it is to embrace spiritual issues. I also think some people don't really find God until they're knocked onto their knees by something. Usually, it's in the hospital when people really develop a relationship with God. Because when things are good, it's easy to forget why they're good."

"So now with this knowledge, what tools can regular people who haven't had a near death experience try to incorporate into their daily lives? How should people get started?" I asked.

"If you take a six-month period of time and write down all the weird things that happen – all the coincidences – and then look back on them, I guarantee that you'll look at those experiences and say 'WOW!' Some people will still call them coincidences – even when there's this unbelievable pattern that would be statistically impossible. I think stories like mine do have the power to help change people because I'm a scientist, which gives me credibility. But I wish people would write things down as they happen. Because it's only when you see God working in your life that you truly can transform faith into trust. Commit to seeing with open eyes. Even if it's three minutes a day – take the time to think about your spiritual life."

At this point I have to lean in to hear Mary's words because the women on Maury are now beating people up in the audience.

"BEEP BEEP BEEP BEEEEEEEEEEEEEEEEEEEEEEEEEEEEEE EEP!!!"

Are Pete and Mary deaf? How can they not be annoyed by this?

It took every amount of focus I had to concentrate on Mary's words rather than the violence on the TV screen.

"You find pennies in the street; you know how it says 'in God we Trust'? When I see a coin in the street, I pick it up and I look at it and I think, 'OK, at this moment in time in my life, am I putting my trust in GOD?' Little things like that. For me at least, I feel I'm continually in prayer all day."

Mary had a calmness about her that was impressive.

I'll have what she's having ...

There was an Oprah series called "Pray the Gay Away". It got me thinking: maybe I could "Pray the Maury Away"?

Thank you in advance, universe, for the blackout, so I don't have to listen to this crap on the TV for one more second.

Then it hit me. For some reason I was supposed to be interviewing Mary next to a blaring television. Not so the guests on Maury could teach me how to open up a can of "whoop-ass" in public, but because I needed a good lesson in spiritual wisdom. There will always be something that distracts you or tempts you to get off the spiritual path.

Don't let Maury Povich take this positive moment away from you, Jen!

"As recently as 2011, 92 percent of all Americans said they believed in God," Mary continued. "Much of the press would like to claim that God is dead; that spirituality is dead. I find that the more complex our society becomes, the more we seek spirituality. I think there's this core inside of us that wants to connect and reconnect. You can try to fill that void with drugs, alcohol, sex, sports. You can try to fill it with a lot of things, but that longing is still there. I try to encourage people to deepen their spirituality a little bit at a time because ultimately, that's the most important thing."

Deepening your spirituality is the most important thing...

⚜ ⚜ ⚜

I walked Mary to the front lobby to say our "goodbyes".

"I'm so grateful for this conversation," I said.

"It was really great to meet you," she said.

We hugged, I felt like no one has hugged me with more sincerity. It was firm, purposeful, and completely full of love. I'd just met this chick and I didn't want to let her go.

As I walked to the elevator, there was a penny on the floor. I never see pennies. Or if I did, I never cared to notice.

I picked it up and read the words: "In God We Trust" and thought of what Mary had told me.

"At this moment in time, am I putting my trust in God?"

We have a choice: we can either be the Mary's of this world or we can be the Maury's.

The only thing standing between heaven and hell is "u".

❦   ❦   ❦

When I got back to my desk, I pitched Mary's story to my editors for a column.

I heard nothing in return.

Am I putting my trust in God?

Usually, it takes several interviews, a few books, and then some serious reflecting for someone's words of wisdom to stick. But just one hour with a lady who got kicked out of heaven was enough to change my perspective. After our conversation, I seemed to have a more conscious way of being, even during those mundane moments that fill up a day. If I were stuck in traffic, I would remind myself to "trust the tapestry". If an assignment seemed annoying or beneath me, I would assume there was someone I was meant to meet in the process. When I'd get ready for work in the morning I would say, "Thank you in advance, universe, for showing me the next steps for my highest good and the highest good of all involved."

Soon, I received an email from the program director from WGN Radio.

"Any chance you can host a show on Mother's Day?" He wrote.

I would have three hours of radio to fill and Dr. Mary Neal was the first guest I booked.

❦   ❦   ❦

Mother's Day morning, I awoke to the sounds of my sad, feverish child standing next to my bed.

"Mommy, I'm going to have a big spit," he said, which was his way of saying a bucket of vomit was in his future. It was 5:20 a.m.

After puking and getting cleaned up, Britt crawled into bed with me as I tickled his back. The alarm wouldn't be sounding for another couple of hours. My desire to drift back to sleep was thwarted by my son's need to chat.

"Mommy, what is that gold trophy on the shelf in my room?" he asked. My son thinks the Emmy I won back in my television reporting days is pretty, so it's been permanently on display next to his "Cat in the Hat" book.

"I won that for telling stories," I said.

"You tell stories?" he asked.

"Yes," I said.

"In your books?"

"Well, that trophy was for something I did for television."

"Do you tell stories about heaven?"

For a second I wondered if I was still half asleep.

"What did you say?"

"Did you tell stories about heaven to win the trophy?"

We rarely talk about heaven, so his bringing it up seemed a bit odd.

"Not for the trophy," I said. "But I tell stories about heaven in my books."

"Good," Britt said.

Good?

"Why do you think that's good?" I asked.

"I think it's important," he said. "If you tell stories about heaven, it can help people."

I tickled his back for a few more minutes as I tried to think of my next question.

"How do you know about heaven, honey?" I asked.

"From Grandpa and Great-Grandma Virginia," he said, without skipping a beat.

Britt seems to have this ability to see my dead Dad and dead Grandma – a party trick I've never fully understood but always envied. I wrote about it in my second book, and have received several emails and letters from other mothers who have the same "problem" with their children.

"My son never met my mother, yet he talks about her all the time," a woman named Deb wrote. "He even knew her wedding anniversary and all of her favorite songs. We never told my son any of these things. How is this possible?"

Dear Deb,
I have no idea. Good luck with that.
Hugs,
Jen

Britt was born long after both my Dad and Granny died, so I'm not quite sure why he seems to know only things they would know. But I try to be encouraging rather than take my index finger and make circles on the side of my head like any normal person might do when someone says they're talking to dead people.

"I miss them so much," he said.

YOU miss them?

"You get to talk to them all the time, hun," I said.

"But it's not the same," he said. "They float so I can't hug them."

Britt often described seeing my Dad and Granny "in the air". From Christmas, to shopping at the Jewel, they visited him frequently. He's even described their outfits in full detail, and my Granny's jewelry, down to the colors of her rings and earrings.

"When was the last time you saw them?" I asked.

"When you were playing the piano yesterday," he said. I had stopped taking piano lessons at the age of 15, but started up again after I bought myself a piano. It was my divorce present. (Some women buy themselves jewelry or clothes. I get a piano.)

"They love when you play, Mom."

My Dad played the piano every night when I was a child. He could play anything – from The Beatles to Chopin. My Granny sang professionally with Vaughn Monroe and his orchestra. Music was a big part of their lives and mine.

I reached for a tissue on the nightstand to wipe my eyes.

"Why are you crying?" Britt asked.

"Because sometimes, I wish Grandpa and Great Grandma Virginia could talk to me too," I said.

Britt turned toward me and looked me right in my sleepy eyes.

"They *do* talk to you, Mommy. You just don't listen."

Oh no he didn't!!

"I don't listen, huh?" I said.

Britt shook his head "no."

I'd spent more time and money over the years taking every spiritual class or seminar you can imagine – from "how to meditate" to "listen to your inner wisdom". And now my kid was telling me I don't listen?

I listen, dammit!!

I took the tissue and blew my nose. I then plopped back onto the pillow and resumed my tickling position.

"You know, I'm going to be talking to a woman today when I go to work who went to heaven," I said.

"What?" Britt said, opening his eyes like saucers.

"Yes, this lady was in a bad accident and she went to heaven, and then the angels told her she couldn't stay because she had to come back to earth and tell everyone her story about heaven so she can help people," I said.

Britt immediately stopped sucking on his fingers and sat up.

"You gotta be kiddin' me!" he gasped.

"I mean it," I said.

Britt fell back onto the pillow with a smile, and put his fingers back in his mouth.

"I KNEW it!" He said.

⚜ ⚜ ⚜

The radio gig went very well. The interview with Mary was one of the best segments of the show. I received lots of emails from listeners who were moved by her story, asking me for more information about her book.

Thank you in advance, universe, for another opportunity to do radio.

Later that day, I stopped by my friend Beth's house for dinner. She is a divorced mother of two. There were three beautiful bouquets on her table that were given to her for Mother's Day. Two were from family and one was just dropped off with a card that said "Love".

"I have no clue who sent that one," She said, genuinely confused. She was not dating, so this floral arrangement was quite the mystery. "Nobody is copping to it."

Why can't I get a mystery bouquet?

I realized this was the first Mother's Day since my marriage that I didn't receive roses. It's not like I thought my ex-husband should spring for a dozen roses. (OK, maybe I did – I mean we were getting along pretty well and I know lots of divorced couples who still take their kid to buy a Father's/Mother's Day gift, saying it's from the kid. Why couldn't my ex be like those people?)

Divorce seems to magnify the loneliness that surrounds all those stupid Hallmark holidays.

When I was getting ready for bed later that night, I started talking to the sky.

"I know I don't need a significant other to make me feel better here, but help me not feel so alone, Dad. Angels. Whomever. If somebody up there hears me and isn't too busy, would you help me not feel so alone?"

❧ ❧ ❧

The following morning, I was working at my desk when I got a call from the Security Guard at the front entrance.

"A woman is down here in the lobby for you," he said.

At that moment I heard a woman grab the phone away from the security guard. She then started blurting into the receiver, "Jenniffer, I have something I'd like to give you."

"Who is this?" I asked.

"Hollis," she said.

Hollis is a friend I'd met recently through work. She was also a good friend of one of my co-workers and she'd read both of my books.

"I'll be right down," I said.

When I got to the lobby, I saw Hollis standing there holding a beautiful bouquet of flowers.

"Who are those for?" I asked.

"These are for you!"

Not only was Hollis holding flowers, FOR ME, but they were my all-time favorite flowers on the planet: pale peach roses.

"These are my favorite flowers," I whispered, barely able to believe my eyes.

"I had to give them to you because you gave me the best gift yesterday," Hollis said.

"I gave YOU a gift? What was that?"

"Your radio show made my day. I gardened yesterday and listened to your entire show and it was so wonderful and inspiring. I'm on my way to radiation treatment right now; but I have to tell you, you gave me the best Mother's Day."

Hollis had recently been diagnosed with breast cancer. While the prognosis looked good she was still recovering from her first surgery.

"I just hope they have you back on the radio soon," she said. "You should have your own show. I am telling you people are hungry for this. I am starving for that kind of a show. You are really tapping into something here – spirituality and a sense of humor and... oh it was just exactly what I needed yesterday. Thank you so much."

My eyes welled up.

"No, thank YOU," I said, giving her a hug.

As I took my flowers up to my desk, I had a big smile on my face.

I thought back to Mary Neal's words, and how she said the best thing we can do is keep a journal and write down all the coincidences or weird things that happen to us that would be impossible to prove.

"I wish people would write things down as they happen. Because it's only when people see God working in their life that they truly can transform faith into trust. Commit to seeing with open eyes and spend the time doing it. Even if it's three minutes a day. Take the time to think about your spiritual life."

Could God really be working in my life? (Especially when she knows how much I swear?!)

⚜ ⚜ ⚜

CHAPTER SIX
WISDOM FROM
AN $800 PAIR OF SHOES

Facebook Status:

Heard on Michigan Avenue- "Just because he was nice to the waiter, doesn't make him an exceptional human being"

✤ ✤ ✤

Have you ever met someone who seems so together, you wonder, "How can this person have it SO together?"

Then you get "together-envy" and sort of wish you had their life?

This is how I felt about my friend Anna. Anna has beautiful red hair and ivory white skin.

Her kids are adorable and her husband is uber successful. Whether she's writing books or transforming schools, she's the kind of person who gets stuff done.

One day after work I was standing on the street and Anna walked by, looking gorgeous. I hadn't seen her in over a year.

"How are you?" I asked.

"Well, I'm totally in hell actually, how about you?" she said.

I thought she was kidding.

"Hey, me too!" I laughed. "Divorce, moving and everything else in between."

"You too?" She said.

What? What do you mean me too?

"You're getting divorced?" I gasped. "No!"

This will totally screw up my idea of someone having everything. Dammit!

We made plans to meet for an appetizer after work a few weeks later. But weeks turned into months and I got so busy with my own chaos, getting together with friends fell to the bottom of the priority list. And then one day Anna reached out in need of a chat.

"How about tomorrow?" I wrote.

"Deal. See you then," she responded.

We met at a restaurant near my job. She looked beautiful as always, but I could tell her heart was heavy with grief.

"My husband moved out, started partying late into the night and seeing younger women," she started to explain. "He came back after about a month of this and decided he wanted to work on our marriage. So we went to therapy but it wasn't helping. Then I get a call two weeks later from his mother who was at my house. She says 'you need to pick up the children right now. The kids are barricaded in the bathroom!' Police were called. It was crazy. My husband had a bi-polar meltdown. He thought he was the CEO of Yahoo. The computer was wrapped up in duct tape. I rescued the kids, pulled them out of there, got restraining orders. And then I got my husband committed. So my descent into hell has been very real. It has taken months just to get my kids back on track."

We ordered some cheese and Anna paused to sip her wine.

"I walked away from my old house and got situated in an apartment. I went to get some cash out of the bank one day and there was nothing in the account," she said. "I'd taken my kids on vacation, and we were driving and I had no way of getting gas. And it's not like you can call people and say, 'oh by the way, my vacation isn't working out – how would you feel about bank rolling us to get home?' My husband had taken total control of our finances. I had no credit. I had not paid a bill in 15 years. I moved into my new place and I got turned down by the cable company. Do you know how low you have to be to get turned down by Comcast?"

Hearing Anna's story, I was so grateful that my ex and I didn't have any of these issues. But I was finding out that my situation was hardly commonplace.

The cheese arrived and Anna started eating – a lot – which was not her usual style.

"So how have you been making ends meet?" I asked.

"The reality is ... I am on food stamps," she whispered. "I am out with people who will drop 400 dollars on dinner and I can't afford soup. It's not like I can eat my shoes – so I have sold a third of my clothes. I sold my engagement ring. Everyone has their own lawyers – the kids, me, him. For the last several months I have been to court every week. I've drained my 401K. It costs $4,000 for three lawyers to show up in court. And as they talk to me I see pictures of my children with things flying away, like their braces – just evaporating. There goes camp. There goes college."

There was one piece of cheese sitting on the plate. Anna reached for it and put it on the remaining piece of bread.

"I've been eating out of food pantries since August," she said.

Anna told the story in such a matter-of-fact tone, it was almost comical – like she was a guest giving a play-by-play on the Jay Leno Show.

"A Jewish food pantry even paid my electric bills and bought Hannukah presents for my kids. The second time I was there, they let me go in the back with a garbage bag. The food donated by upper middle class Jews is fabulous. My kids could live on capers and Carr's Water Crackers until the Messiah returns."

Anna had lost everything except her sense of humor.

"And this has given me a tremendous insight. I mean, do you know how impossible it is to get food stamps? I have a PhD and it's impossible! It's like this club where they make it incredibly difficult to break into the system." (She paused to sip her wine.)

"Nobody picks up the phone at any of these places. You have to go there at 8 a.m. and you're there with this sea of humanity. The first three times I went I couldn't get an appointment to talk with someone. It's so tragic."

"Does your ex not realize that by taking this all out on you he's hurting your children?" I asked.

"I'm the target now of all his rage," she said. "Yet this happened because he didn't want to be married anymore and wanted to go clubbing. Still, I'm the bad guy. It's so insane."

Anna shook her head as the waitress approached our table.

"Would you like some more?"

I could see Anna's hesitation.

"Bring us another cheese platter. This is on me," I smiled.

"In that case, can I get another wine?" Anna asked with a laugh.

"Coming right up," said the waitress.

"I have this funny food stamps story," Anna continued as she nibbled on her bread. "A friend of mine from New York sent me a pair of $800 Chanel ballet flats."

"What?" I gasped.

"I know. I need $800 shoes like I need a hole in the head. Incredibly sweet gesture; but that would pay half my rent. So you know what? These Chanel ballet flats are my power shoes that tell me I'm not supposed to be this broken girl forever. They're magical. I'm wearing them now."

I looked down and saw a gorgeous pair of sparkling ballet flats.

"So that's what $800 shoes look like," I joked.

"I wore these when I went for the fourth time to get my emergency food stamps that I have been awarded but can't seem to get an appointment to actually receive regularly! So I'm waiting in line ... and the man next to me has a seizure."

"No!"

"Yes. He collapsed onto the floor."

"Oh my God! What did you do?"

"Well, it then became clear that he was going to be alright, which is good of course, but he had frothed all over my shoes," she said.

I couldn't remember the last time I'd heard the word "frothed".

"On your $800 dollar shoes?"

"I couldn't make this shit up! So I thought, that's perfect. If they were going to get ruined, of course they would get ruined by a person dying for food stamps. And because I am such a JAP, all I can think is, oh my God, because this guy had a seizure, everyone has cleared out and now there's no line. I'm gonna get seen today!"

Anna's second glass of wine came, as well as the cheese.

"I haven't eaten this well or had good wine in so long," she said. I could see her savoring every bite and sip.

"So you got your stamps, and you're getting by," I said. "Do you have any contact now with the ex?"

"Oh you won't believe this," she said. "He wants me back."

"What?!"

"He says he's sorry and he knows he messed up the one thing that was best in the world. It threw me into a quandary of wondering: if things were to go back to normal, would I want him back? And the truth is, a lot has happened over this time. I'm not the same person. I am now forever altered, and not in very good ways either.

I couldn't imagine looking at him and thinking he's cute or sexy. Or respecting him or having faith in him or believing in him – or believing in us. I don't even think I could watch him eat anymore without being disgusted. Anything that was a foible or annoying behavior is now so magnified, because you overlook all of this stuff when you're together and it's all part of the fiction of marriage. I don't think I could love him that way again. To me, nothing else matters except keeping my kids on an emotional even keel. They are the most important thing."

"How are they doing?" I asked.

"They're getting there," she said. "We have a really great support system at their school. And I have been weeping with my friends, who have been so kind. All of my friends – everyone – has pitched in. Yesterday someone sent me groceries. Anything anyone could do, they have done. I had friends in rotation who would call me every three hours."

"It's funny, but the people I least expected to get help from have showed up for me and the ones I expected to be there disappeared," I said, referring to my own divorce. "One of my oldest friends shut me off completely. I think she's afraid she's going to 'catch' a divorce."

"There is no shame in saying, 'I need help!' Anna said. "If friends don't respond, they don't. But you have to ask. We think we have to do everything ourselves in a crisis and guess what, we can't. We fucking can't. And that's OK."

Anna's words were still soaking in as the waitress brought more water.

"You know, I might just go ahead and reach out to some girlfriends later," I said.

"Oh, I got the BEST email the other day from a friend of mine," she said, jumping out of her seat. "You have to hear this." Anna pulled out her phone and began to read. "Everyone could learn from this woman. This is the email to send out when you end a marriage."

"I did the dirty deed. I ended it. Finally. Now, I need massive amounts of love and support because I don't have as hard of a time breaking up with him as I do staying broken up. There's a sneaky feeling that pops up that it will never get better than this. My brain picks it up and runs with it. I feel like it's my fault that it didn't work – that if I'd just tried harder... I need some serious sunlight to shine on that untrue fact. The universe, the Goddess, someone, has something better in store for me, right? So what can you do? Call me, email, text me, visit me, or I will visit you. Remind me that even if I'm alone it is better, MUCH better than what I was doing. Tell me that I am young and interesting and that lots of cool shit will happen to me in my life, and that ending it with this man frees me up to see it. And anything else that you can think of – like buy me vegan raw food cookbooks and trips to Cozumel. No wait, how about letting me make YOU dinner and macaroons? Anyhow, thank you for being the women in my life who have my metaphorical back. Love, Melanie."

"I think I need to go home and write an email," I said, feeling my pride give way to reality.

"Do it," she said. "My friends are the only way I'm getting through this."

⚜ ⚜ ⚜

When I got home, I pulled out the laptop and wrote a note to a handful of friends asking for emotional support. But each time I tried to hit "send" I would panic. I realized that asking for help was not part of my skill set. In my world you figure it out on your own. You don't reach out to others.

You can do this, Jen. You deserve this.

I finally sent off the email and took a deep breath.

"Asking for help is not a sign of weakness," I remembered my therapist telling me. "It shows great strength to express your needs. And don't assume those close to you can read your mind either."

Never assume.

Wisdom can be delivered in many different packages. And on this day, it showed up for me in an $800 dollar pair of shoes.

⚜   ⚜   ⚜

Chapter Seven
Sometimes We Need to Get Drunk on a Wayne-Anita Cocktail

Facebook Status:

Heard on Michigan Avenue: "Do you think God would forgive me if he knew how selfish I was?"

"He knows, Dennis. And he loves you anyway."

❧ ❧ ❧

The morning I was supposed to interview Wayne Dyer for the radio I was really in a funk.

"I'm kinda crabby today, Mary," I warned my co-host. "I need a cookie or something."

I reached into my purse to see if there was anything resembling something sweet. I was hoping for a spare piece of chocolate, but all I found were three of my son's matchbox cars and several pens.

Mary saw my struggle and pulled out a small container.

"Mint?" she offered.

Altoids did not appeal nearly as much as a cookie.

"No thanks," I said.

"How was your date last night?" she asked.

"He rubbed Purell on my hand before shaking it," I said, dropping my head onto the table.

"What?!"

"Yeah. He wouldn't shake my hand until he'd sanitized it."

"What is wrong with people?"

"I've got Wayne on the line," our producer said through the speakers. "We're coming up in about a minute."

In the eyes of my mother, Wayne Dyer is the closest thing on this earth to God. While I don't quite put him in this category, the guy has over 30 books under his belt and enough PBS specials to keep my mom permanently tuned in, so he's obviously doing something right. I have read many of his books. My favorite is "There's a Spiritual Solution to Every Problem." What really draws me to Wayne is that he's open about his struggles with alcohol, his battle with cancer, and his separation from his wife. No topic is off limits. This guy doesn't claim to be perfect. He shows us how human he is in his journey to find enlightenment.

"Please refer to him as DOCTOR Dyer," his handler told us before the interview took place.

I wondered why the hell a spiritual teacher who claims that all living beings are "children of God" needed to be referred to by a title.

That's not very spiritual.

"We're back in 30," the producer said through our headphones.

Thank you in advance, universe, for Wayne Dyer saying something that will help turn my frown upside down.

The commercials ended and it was time to perk up.

"Welcome back to WGN-Radio, the voice of Chicago. I'm Jenniffer Weigel with my co-host Mary Long, and we're very excited to introduce our special guest who's calling us all the way from his home in Hawaii: Dr. Wayne Dyer," I said.

"It's lovely to speak with you ladies," Dyer said.

"Thank you Dr. Dyer," said Mary.

As Wayne started chatting about "Mastering the Art of Manifestation", the phone lines lit up.

"I keep putting things into my imagination and nothing is changing for me," one caller said.

"Real success comes through service and gratitude," said Wayne. "I don't have a vision board with a new Mercedes or a new watch on it. I wake up each day and ask, 'what can I give?' The first thing I do every single morning is say, 'thank you.' Then I'll pick a letter up, or sometimes I'll call someone. I try to give back. I ask, 'how may I serve somebody?"

Now I was confused. Much of Wayne's message revolves around putting what you want into your imagination. This is similar to the "vision board" way of thinking: if you think it and wish it to be so, you can make it happen.

"Things come to you when you give to others," he said.

"One of your mantras is, 'I'm healthy, I'm happy, I'm wealthy'; but many struggle to get that wealth piece," Mary said.

"Wealth isn't about the dollars in your pocket. It's about the love in your heart," he said. "Our relationships with ourselves and with others need to be rich and wealthy. That is true wealth."

"Wayne, how do you coach people when the economy is down and people are feeling hopeless?" I asked.

Oh crap –I called him Wayne!

"You have to create opportunities for yourself, Jenniffer. When I was in the orphanage I shoveled snow or delivered papers because I wanted some spending money, but nobody would give it to me. A lot of people have a sense of entitlement that somebody else ought to do these things for them. People are mad at the government for not getting jobs for them. I don't understand why it's the government's responsibility. Jobs are disappearing because the world is changing. If you live in a town and the factory is closed, you can't just sit there and hope that the factory comes back. You might have to move. You have to adjust to the world that you live in. And we only need so much to survive; but this world we live in tells us we need more stuff to be happy. We're inundated with our televisions, the internet and advertising that tell us in order to be happy we have to have these things. When you say, 'gimme, gimme, gimme,' you will always be in short supply. But if you ask, 'how may I serve?' things will come to you. You attract who you are." "Dr. Dyer, you talk a lot about the ego and how it can block things from manifesting. Can you explain?" Mary asked.

"The ego makes us think we are separate from each other and therefore special. But we are not," he said. "So if you go through your

108

day thinking you are better than someone else or more worthy of success, you completely disconnect from source. You are competing and thinking you are special. And this prevents you from bringing in your greatest gifts. When approval-seeking is the guiding principle of life it's virtually impossible to achieve a loving relationship with another human being. We can't give it away to others if we don't have it for ourselves."

"What do you say to skeptics who say this isn't based in science?" I asked.

"The science of today is not the same as the science of 20 years ago," he said. "It's not just what you can see and touch. Now we're told there are these subatomic particles which recognize that all matter is nothing but energy. Science is constantly changing its mind."

"I know the spiritual belief is that you don't need money to be fulfilled, but I'll tell ya, there's something very nice about being able to pay your bills, Wayne!" Mary said.

"Yes, paying your bills is important; but there are some people who never seem to get enough, and when they get a little they need more. It's a cycle that never stops. If you are valuing success based on the accumulation of things, just because you have cars or maybe you're selling books, it doesn't mean you have a connection with God or something greater," he said. "That's the ego. I call that 'edging God out.' You can't call yourself a kind person if you're not kind to the person who cleans your toilet. You have to go to your core – your originating value, source, or God – whatever you want to call it. It's what you came from. We are all love or source. This is who we are ... and once we discover that, then we look at people differently."

Edging god out...

❧ ❧ ❧

A couple of days later, I was sitting at my desk and weeding through my work emails. I receive approximately 20 pitches a day.

"Dear Jenniffer, more and more people are buying vibrators over the counter ..."

Delete.

"Dear Jenniffer, I am writing you today to see if you have any interest in my client's latest invention: Doggie seat belts ..."

Delete.

"Dear Jenniffer, Dr. Dyer really enjoyed the interview with you and Mary over the weekend. He will be coming to Chicago in a couple of weeks."

Now we're talkin'!

A couple of days later, Wayne and I chatted for nearly 45 minutes over the phone and covered everything from his troubling childhood to his divorce. Once I felt comfortable with him I had to ask:

"So your publicist told us that we had to refer to you as Doctor Dyer on the radio. I'm just curious why you would be attached to a title?"

"You're kidding," He said, seemingly shocked. "I couldn't care less about a title. That's all part of the ego. Truly, call me Wayne."

OK Wayne, ole' buddy ole' pal.

"You really are open about how difficult it was for you growing up. Can you tell me more about that?" I asked.

"When I was young my brother David and I were farmed off to foster homes and I spent time in orphanages. My father abandoned us. Here's the most important person in my life and I never met him. I went to his gravesite and I was able to forgive him and get rid of my rage and anger. Until you are able to do that with anyone in your life – whether it's family or a friend or someone you work with – you can't move forward and bring true joy into your life. I have made a clear point in my life to clean up the anxiety, stress, hatred and bitterness. If I were to die in the next hour, there is nobody I haven't forgiven."

"You talk about how you are no longer with your wife, yet you two are making a conscious effort to co-parent and be there for your kids, correct?" I asked.

"Well, at 60 my wife met someone who was almost 30 years her junior," he said in a not-so-spiritual tone. "But she and I talk almost every day. We have seven children together. She lives with another man in the house that I built; and at first I was angry and upset; but it was absolutely necessary."

Your wife shacking up with a dude half her age in the house you built was necessary?!

"When you go through deep struggles – when you come into this world with big darma – big things to do – then you can dig through obstacles. You need to deal with those obstacles instead of dealing with the stuff in complaint ... and use gratitude/ Say to yourself, 'I am grateful.' That's how I feel about the cancer diagnosis and our separation. You dig through the obstacles. My wife and I are closer than we have ever been. We care about each other deeply."

"You mentioned the cancer diagnosis. How is that going?" I asked.

"I am well," he said. "Sure, there might be studies or tests that say otherwise, but I am putting it into my imagination that I am healthy. There is a woman named Anita Moorjani who had terminal cancer and she was on her deathbed. She had a near-death experience, and while she was in a coma she was told this was 'not her time.' She could see everyone who was working on her in the hospital and she could hear their thoughts. She was in this coma for 30 hours but was in the hospital on death's door for nearly five weeks. When she awoke she was shown that she can heal the cancer in her body and that all cancer is preceded by a cancer in our energy body; and if we heal our energy body then our physical bodies will correspond to it. Nobody has ever come back from cancer at this stage. She has baffled the medical community. She was technically dead. Yet she woke up and she has completely healed. No doctors can explain it. It's the most incredible miracle I have ever come across in my life. I'm writing the forward to her book. You have to talk to her. She is incredibly inspiring."

Immediately after our conversation, I went onto Youtube and watched several conversations with Anita Moorjani. One quote in particular stood out.

"It's not about pursuing – the minute we talk about pursuing something – the fact that you feel you have to go after it means you don't really think it's yours in the first place. But when you're at that centered place – then everything that is yours just comes to you; you just have to allow it."

I quickly emailed some links of Anita's interviews to a couple of friends I thought needed to hear her the most.

❧ ❧ ❧

The next day I went to lunch with my friend Lisa. Ever since I've known Lisa, she has been trying to write a book. It's been over ten years now, and her book has changed at least eight times. She wanted to meet so she could tell me the new focus and how she planned to get it published.

"I've really got it this time," she said.

She then went on to describe the topics in her book and why she has made so many changes. As she rattled things off, I felt as though I was sitting next to a spinning top that was about to take flight.

Meanwhile – for once in my life – I felt completely calm. It was as if I was drunk on a Wayne-Anita cocktail. When Lisa came up for air, she looked at me for a reaction. I nodded my head and said, "if this is your authentic story, all you have to do is trust that it will wind up in the right hands and the right editor will come to you rather than you going after the right editor," I said. "You have planted the seeds and tended your garden. Now it's time for someone to come and admire your work."

I paused to see if my words were sinking in and got no reaction, so I continued.

"It's not about pursuing. The minute you talk about pursuing something, the fact that you feel you have to go after it means you don't really think it's yours in the first place. But when you're at that centered place, then everything that is yours just comes to you. You just have to allow it."

Lisa looked at me with a frown. Her head sort of cocked to the side like a dog hearing a noise for the first time.

"You seem very sure of yourself," she said.

She was right. I was sure of myself. And I was sure that her way, as it had proven for over a decade, was not getting her the desired results.

"Did you watch that video I sent you of the woman who was in the coma that Wayne Dyer told me about?" I asked.

Lisa blinked her eyes a few times and gave me a blank stare.

"Ok; well, it really changed my life. I mean, it totally sunk in for me," I said. "The universe needs everyone. All you have to do is be your authentic self and everything will fall into place."

Have you ever discovered something that you found to be so valuable that you want to shout it from the rooftops? But when you try to suggest to someone else to give it a whirl, they run in the other direction?

We ate our food in silence for a minute.

"This woman, Anita, said that our need to constantly go after things and reach outside of ourselves actually prevents us from getting what is divinely ours. It's almost as if it resets the GPS when you make a wrong turn during a long drive. You still might eventually get there, but it just takes a little bit longer," I said.

The visual I use for Anita's words is this: when you are vacuuming the rug in the living room, and you try to stretch the cord just a little too far to do the dining room, the power cord isn't long enough and it pops out of the wall. The moment you reach too far outside of yourself, the cord comes unplugged, and you are literally unplugged from the power source.

Lisa picked at her food.

"I have seen you struggle with this for so long," I said. "I just really want to see you succeed. And all these changes because of this person or that person ... there are too many cooks in the kitchen. Just write your story and trust that it will get published. Put in the work and create your story, and then let it go."

We continued to eat and I tried to lighten the mood.

"Do you want to come with me to see Wayne Dyer and about 800 of his closest friends?" I asked.

"No thanks," she said.

"When you are totally being yourself, all you can be is love because that's who you are at your core – so don't be afraid to be who you are."

-Anita Moorjani

❧ ❧ ❧

A few nights later, Mary and I went to Wayne's event.

The room was packed. As we settled into our seats, I looked down at my blackberry and there was an email from Wayne.

"Be sure to approach the stage when you arrive," he wrote. "I want to say hello to you in person."

OMG! My new friend, Wayne Dyer, wants to say hello!

"Wayne said to approach the stage to say hello before the talk," I said to Mary.

"Great!" she said.

As he walked into the room, several people were making their way up to him to get his autograph.

"Let's go!" Mary said.

"I don't want to hound him," I said, sitting back down in my chair. "He has a line of people there."

"He said to approach, so let's approach," she said.

We slowly walked toward the stage and waited as the group thinned out. I felt a bit awkward. I also felt the glare of 800 people burning a hole in the back of my head.

"Who does she think she is?"

Wayne was taller than I expected, and had a booming voice as he addressed every single person with complete focus. As I got closer, I noticed his smile, which I found to be very authentic and soothing. He wore a beret and black turtleneck – sort of a "high school drama teacher" vibe. After what felt like a lifetime, it was finally our turn to say "hello."

"Hi Wayne – we are Jen and Mary from WGN Radio," I said.

He hugged each of us and then put his arm on my shoulder.

"It is so nice to meet you both," he said.

I have no idea what came out of my mouth for the next couple of minutes. I felt like I'd morphed into a teenage version of myself trying to talk to the popular boy at the school dance. Then before I knew it, it was time to sit down.

"Have a great show," Mary said, cueing our exit.

"Thanks to you both," he said.

Wayne's talk lasted nearly three hours. When I got home to relieve the babysitter, I sent him a "gratitude" email.

"Your work is changing lives. Thank you for doing what you do," I wrote.

⚜ ⚜ ⚜

As I sat at my desk the following day, I received an email from Wayne.

"Call me at my hotel ..."

I had to rub my eyes to make sure I wasn't hallucinating.

Wayne Dyer wants me to call him? At his hotel??!

I slowly picked up the phone and dialed. I didn't know why but my heart was racing.

Why would Wayne Dyer want to talk to me?

I dialed the number, asked for his room number and he picked up the phone.

"Hello?" he said.

"Yes, I'd like to place an order," I said.

Long pause.

"An order?" he asked.

"Yes, with the universe," I continued. "I'm looking for eternal happiness and everlasting bliss. And that's for here, please."

Wayne let out a big belly laugh.

"Well, all you have to do is put it in your imagination," he said.

After some small talk Wayne invited me to dinner with his family, which included his brother, who lived in Chicago, and his daughter.

"I would love to, Wayne. But I have a book talk tonight," I said.

Son of a bitch!

Yes, Wayne Dyer just invited me to dinner, and I had a previous commitment. I was going to be chatting to a group at a Catholic Church. There was actually a bit of a controversy about my impending talk. Since one of my books is titled, "I'm Spiritual, Dammit!", some people wondered if my presence in the church was appropriate. They took white-out to the posters announcing my event. I was the author of "I'm Spiritual ......" I found it very ironic that a group who claims to love Jesus could literally judge a book by its cover.

Why did I have to say "yes" to this Catholic group?

"If there was a way to be both places at once, Wayne, I would be there in a second," I said.

"Just put that into your imagination too," he joked.

"OK, I'll give it a shot," I said. "If it works and I'm able to time travel, I'll see you at dinner."

"I look forward to it," he said.

Within seconds of hanging up with Wayne I called my mother.

"Mom, I just had to turn Wayne Dyer down for dinner," I said, trying to keep my voice down at my cubicle.

"What?" She gasped. "What do you have to do that is more important than dinner with Wayne Dyer?" She asked.

"I'm doing a book talk at a church," I said.

"And you can't cancel? They'd understand, wouldn't they?"

"No, it's too late," I said. "The talk is in three hours."

"I'm proud of you for honoring your commitment," she said. "Maybe there will be another chance to have a dinner with Wayne. Where does he live?"

"Hawaii."

"Oh well."

⚜ ⚜ ⚜

As I pulled up to the talk, I was nervous for some reason. Knowing that some of the parents were anxious over the title of my book, I wondered how much I'd have to change so I wouldn't offend the crowd. I had to center myself in the car before walking into the church.

You are where you're supposed to be in every moment; and tonight, someone in this church needs to hear you speak. Otherwise you would be having dinner with Wayne Dyer and his family. Right? This is meant to be. Right? RIGHT? Just tell your stories from your heart. Be yourself.

And for heaven's sake, don't say "fuck".

I got a box of books out of my trunk and made my way into the building. They had an area set up behind the main building for me, complete with several adult beverages and a variety of home-made snacks. The woman who organized the event greeted me right away.

"We are *so* glad you are here," she cooed.

"Wow, you guys thought of everything!" I said, looking at several wine bottles lining the table.

"We like to drink," she laughed. "Help yourself to anything."

This church is located directly behind the house where I first lived as a child. Eventually, the room started filling up, and I felt like it was an episode of "This Is Your Life." Everyone – from old neighbors to babysitters – came to hear me talk. There were also two priests present.

Two priests, a babysitter and your neighbor walked into a bar ...

If I could win over this bunch, I could do anything.

Thank you in advance, universe, for having me tell whatever stories this group needs to hear. May my words help to heal and inspire.

❧   ❧   ❧

Driving home, I felt at peace. As I pulled into my garage, I remembered what Wayne had said about putting things into your imagination to make them happen. I took a deep breath and tried to imagine I was arriving just in time for dessert with Wayne and his family.

You are with Wayne Dyer. You are with Wayne Dyer.

I pictured us ordering some sort of chocolate cake that would arrive with several forks so we could all share. There was laughter and stimulating conversation. After a few minutes, I opened my eyes.

Apparently my teleporting skills needed more work because I was still in my garage.

When I entered the house, I got the dog's leash and took him for a walk. As Max and I were descending the porch stairs, I heard something in the bushes. There are so many cats in my neighborhood I wasn't scared at all – until I saw the white stripe on top of the black body.

Oh shit. A skunk.

I flashed back to the last time I had to deal with the funk of a skunk. It was 13 years ago and I was at my Dad's house for a dinner party. His cocker spaniel, Burt, had gotten out of the yard, only to return with a sheepish grin and a terrible stench.

"Get some tomato juice!" someone yelled.

We didn't have tomato juice – just spicy Bloody Mary mix. So we dragged Burt into the bathtub and dumped a couple of bottles of Mrs. T's Spiciest all over him. His scent was back to normal, eventually. (Although we were picking pepper flakes out of his fur for weeks.)

So here I was back in present time with my dog, Max, hoping to God we didn't suffer the same fate. (My kitchen was devoid of any tomato juice and I'd killed the Bloody Mary mix a couple of weeks ago.)

I once heard that skunks really don't want to spray you. This is just what happens when *they* get scared. Whether or not it's true, my dog didn't seem alarmed at all. The skunk stopped as my dog continued to sniff the bushes. They were now about five feet from each other, and I slowly pulled Max's leash closer to my side without making any sudden movements. We started walking again as the skunk followed. He stayed closer to the houses while we remained on the sidewalk, but he was practically matching Max's stride.

Oh my God. Oh my God. Don't panic. Everything's fine.

As I got a good look at him, he was actually sort of cute. He waddled a little bit as he walked, which made him more endearing. I could just picture the skunk talking to me if he were a character in a Pixar movie.

"I'm so misunderstood, Jen. I just don't have any real friends ... Can't we all just get along?"

Sigh.

We walked for a block, although it felt more like five miles, and I thought about the symbolism of this "skunk" stroll. What if we chose this kind of tolerance and calm for everything that scared the shit out of us? Whether it's a boss or a Newt Gingrich fan, shouldn't we just be able to walk side-by-side without spraying each other? We are all unique – some of us are smelly and some of us are not, but we all have a place and a purpose. Can't we share the street and maybe even find something we like about that scary thing that's making our heart race with anxiety?

Can't we?

I made it home, and the skunk watched as I walked up the stairs to my front door. My dog lifted his leg for the 500th time on a different bush before following behind me and retiring for the night.

I smiled as I took my dog's leash off.

I walked with a skunk and I'm still OK.

Even the things we assume will do the most damage could turn out to be totally harmless. All we have to do is approach them with a calm, neutral attitude.

As I dozed off to sleep, I pictured putting things into my imagination as Wayne recommended.

I'm healthy, I'm happy, I'm wealthy … I'm healthy, I'm happy, I'm wealthy …

⚜ ⚜ ⚜

CHAPTER EIGHT
THANK YOU, JESUS

Facebook Status:

I did a book talk today. One of the women said she would pray for my soul because my book is called "I'm Spiritual, Dammit!" I told her if my book title was sending me to hell she may want to forget about it. I might be a lost cause.

⚜ ⚜ ⚜

One day at work, I was going through emails.

Hey Jen-
Have you heard about the book "The Boy Who Came Back From Heaven"?

My friend Jan had a new book suggestion.

Nope. Good?

You would love it. I'm going to give it to you today.

Later, we met for lunch and she handed me the book.

"I seriously read it in a day," she said.

I looked down at the title.

"'A true story by Alex and Kevin Malarkey.'" I read. "I'm supposed to believe a 'true story' by the Malarkey's?"

"It's a father and son who both died in a car accident. The son remembers being in heaven. It's fascinating," Jan said.

What's with all this heaven stuff?

We sat there for a minute sipping our tea. We'd both recently decided to take on "The Master Cleanse," which basically means you sip lemonade made with lemon juice, cayenne pepper and maple syrup for ten days straight. No meat, no sugar, no dairy, no caffeine, no booze, no carbs – nothing for ten days except lemonade.

While some people do this to lose weight, I was doing it to flush out my system of toxins. I'd been eating a steady stream of ched-dar cheese and processed food for months and was feeling very unhealthy. Jan had done the cleanse successfully the year before and said it gave her incredible energy.

We were on day three. I was ready to gnaw off my arm.

"Want some gum?" she asked, popping a piece of Trident into her mouth.

"I thought we were trying to rid our bodies of toxins and you're asking me if I want sugar-free gum filled with chemicals?" I laughed.

"It's the closest thing I've had to food in three days," she said. "I need to chew on something."

I found it interesting that when I announced I'd be doing this cleanse to friends and family, some tried to talk me out of it and oth-ers tried to get me to cheat. Most thought it was not only unhealthy but many told me it was unrealistic. I came to realize that when you do something really challenging (like a cleanse or maybe a marathon) it brings up in others all those things they wish they had the courage to do themselves.

I was excited about the thought of flushing all the crud I'd ingested out of my bowels with a steady diet of vitamin C and Cayenne pepper, but I was getting really weak.

"I sat at my computer and read the same sentence four times today," I said to Jan. "I have no concentration. Did you have that problem?"

"I don't remember," she said.

That would be a "yes."

"The first four days are the hardest," she said. "After you get over the hump it gets easier."

That night I watched my son eat cheese pizza. I never realized what a garbage disposal I was during my kid's meals until I was no longer allowed to eat off his plate.

My dog Max got very plump during my cleanse.

I put the kettle on the stove and made myself some hot tea. As I cut my lemon I started fantasizing about lemon pie; lemon smoothies; lemon cake. Anything of substance that included lemons that wasn't that damn juice with a shake of Cayenne pepper and maple syrup.

I hate you, maple syrup.

The following day, I was going on television for my weekly segment where I talk about my column. As I was sitting in the makeup chair, I felt dizzy.

"Are you OK?" One of the other anchors asked.

"I'm doing this cleanse and it's starting to piss me off," I barked. "I'll be fine."

I barely remember what came out of my mouth for my segment on the news, but as I was walking off the set a chef who had just prepared a dish for the cooking segment was handing out extra portions to the crew.

Of COURSE they have food on the show today. SHIT!

The entree involved some sort of spicy meat that smelled so incredibly good I could have injured someone to have just one bite.

"You want a taste?" the chef asked, dishing out plates.

"No thanks," I said, walking away in defeat.

Toxins. Remember I'm flushing out toxins. There's a glass of lemonade in my future. Can't wait!

I got in my car and took a deep breath. My usual routine after a segment on the noon news was to grab a turkey sandwich at a local deli before making the fifteen-minute drive back to my office.

You can do this, Jen. You're only on day four!

The thought of depriving myself for six more days without nutrition seemed completely impossible.

Pizza. What I wouldn't do for a slice of pizza.

I quickly snapped out of my food fantasies when I noticed a car parked on the wrong side of the street facing oncoming traffic. This was on a very busy intersection and the woman driving the car was just sitting in the driver's seat, hands on the steering wheel, not moving.

Is she drunk?

I pulled over, parked, and got out of my car to see if she was OK. As I approached her vehicle I could see she looked very distressed. Traffic heading in her direction had completely stopped and people were starting to honk.

"Are you alright?" I asked. She shook her head "no" and seemed very disoriented. I don't think she'd been drinking but something was definitely not right in her world.

As I took my phone out to call 9-1-1 a police car pulled up with his lights flashing. The large traffic jam now being caused by this woman's decision to park in the wrong lane had obviously gotten his attention.

"What's going on here?" he asked.

"I was just driving and I noticed she was facing oncoming traffic so I got out of the car to see if she was alright," I said.

At this point, the woman was still facing forward with a blank expression on her face. Suddenly, she got out of the car. The policeman reached to put his hand on his gun, unsure of her intentions.

She started walking into traffic. The officer quickly followed her and tried to bring her closer to her car and out of danger. She seemed like she was about to pass out.

"I'm so dizzy," she mumbled.

Maybe she's doing the Master Cleanse too.

As I watched her wander aimlessly on the busy street, it hit me: I wasn't too far off from being in the same sorry shape as this woman. Nutritionally, I was probably one day away from sitting in my Subaru facing the wrong direction. Nobody should be operating heavy machinery in my condition.

Enough of this cleanse bullshit.

The officer took the woman out of harm's way and called for an ambulance. I got back in my car and drove away. No matter how much I wanted to do the liquid diet to flush out my bowels, it wasn't worth putting myself or anyone else at risk.

I hope she'll be OK.

I quickly visualized sending the woman some angels and started driving. I needed food and I needed it fast. While I was tempted to hit the McDonald's drive-through, I decided that rather than shock my system with processed meat and deep fried potatoes, I'd treat myself to some Jamba Juice.

Yes, I broke my cleanse with a fruit smoothie and a shot of wheatgrass.

I'm a criminal.

I sat in my car sipping my liquid meal like a drug addict on the reality show "Intervention" who just sold her mom's jewelry to get a heroin fix. Ten minutes later I had more energy than someone on four cups of coffee.

I pulled out my phone to text Jan, my cleanse buddy.

"I almost hit the drive-through today," I wrote, not fully revealing I'd fallen off the wagon.

"Just had a burrito and a margarita," she wrote back. "I fell hard. They let go of some people in the office today. Rough day. Back on the treadmill tomorrow though."

Meat AND booze?

I decided to continue with a "partial cleanse" for the rest of my ten days. I stayed on the liquids but added protein drinks and smoothies to my diet.

"I cheated today with a 'super-food' smoothie," I said to my co-worker on day six.

"That's not cheating, it's called survival," she said.

That weekend I went up to visit my mother. I figured being closer to nature in Wisconsin would help take my mind off dining out – which was my usual m.o. I took Jan's book with me about the boy who went to heaven in case I felt like cracking it open.

I read it in one sitting.

While the language was a bit too "religious" for me – (the author, Kevin Malarkey, mentions Jesus, God or "The Christian Fellowship" on almost every page) I really was moved by the story. Part of it was that the son, Alex, who died in the car accident but came back to life, was the exact age as my son. Every mention of that boy struggling to stay alive made my eyes well up with tears.

Alex's account of being in heaven was stunning. The power of prayer seemed to really have an impact. But his father's stubborn desire to help his son become "fully recovered" and walk again really bugged me. Not because I don't believe in praying for someone, but because the father thinks a "full recovery" is when his son can climb trees and run on the playground. Alex is still in a wheelchair and he probably always will be. The father's tone of disappointment over this really made me sad. They even got a vanity license plate that says: WIL WALK for inspiration.

He IS fully recovered. Don't you see?

While Alex can't run on the playground, his mind is sharp and his wit is quick. He can love and he can feel and he can talk. He wants to be a comedian as well as a preacher. His family can hold his hand and kiss his face and interact with him everyday. The fact that this is not "fully recovered" in the mind of the dad made my heart ache for Alex. I felt that he had stayed alive for his family. Alex even said he loved going to sleep so he could be with God and Jesus. How can this boy ever feel like he's good enough if his father keeps looking at things with this perspective?

Then there's the whole idea that if you don't belong to their church, you will burn in hell. That was annoying as... well, *hell.*

Besides those two issues, it was a very good book.

Dad Kevin was also very honest in his writings about how his marriage suffered while trying to get their son healthy. Between the task of caring for a boy in a wheelchair to the mounting medical bills, Kevin and his wife, Beth, nearly split up. He talked often of praying with their pastor to save their marriage. "We are told in scripture to keep our eyes on Jesus, even in the midst of a raging storm," he wrote.

I thought about my marriage. My ex and I buried three of our four parents in five years. They each died a slow and painful death from cancer. We managed to make it through all of these hard times, yet we still got divorced.

Maybe if we just prayed harder we would have made it? We should have gone to church more. If we had a pastor who could have made house calls perhaps things would have been different.

My thoughts started to sound like all those assholes who judged my choices when I announced my marriage was ending.

"You made a vow with God as your witness. You can't break that under any circumstances. People just don't try hard enough anymore."

I was envious of the Malarkey's faith in Jesus and in God; but once again their belief that it's "their way or no way" turned me off. This kind of religious faith has a way of ruining religion for the rest of us. I like Jesus – I'm just not a big fan of some of his followers.

The next day I drove home from Wisconsin alone because Britt was with his dad. Driving in solitude was a rare treat. I left the music off and enjoyed the landscape. As I let my mind wander, I thought more and more about Alex's journey to heaven and his time with a being he believed was the spirit of Jesus. I thought about my son, so full of love and faith in angels.

Britt hasn't been baptized. The Malarkey's would say he won't be allowed in heaven. How could a loving God reject an angel like my son because he hasn't been baptized?

I'm more faithful in my spiritual practice than most church-going people I know, yet I couldn't get this dichotomy out of my head. I decided it was time to have a heart-to-heart with a well-known healer named Jesus.

Hey there buddy. I know I haven't chatted with you lately. Been praying to "the universe" rather than to you because to be honest, your name invokes some frustration within me. Chalk it up to my Christian upbringing and some really judgmental Christians I have known through the years. But I have to say I'm a big fan of your work. I know that the essence of who you are is pure love and healing and that you were a pretty amazing dude. I don't want my upbringing to come between us having a decent relationship.

So today, I'm going to try something. I'd like to really open my heart. The most important relationship I can have is with myself. I'm choosing to feel love so I can truly love myself. I can't be in a healthy partnership with another until I'm completely happy with the partnership I have with myself.

So with you as my witness, I ask for love to flow through me.

I sat in silence and felt an incredible warmth come through my body. The top of my head tingled and a sense of peace came over me.

This is awesome.

I pictured my heart filling with light. As I took a few deep breaths, I saw my phone light up out of the corner of my eye. I picked it up and glanced down to find a text message the length of a monologue.

Just pick up the phone and call me!

Still driving, I waited until I pulled over for gas to read the message. It was from my friend Ingrid, with whom I hadn't spoken in a few months.

"Hey, Jen. I've been meaning to ask you for a couple of weeks now. We have a family friend who is dying to meet you. He's divorced with three kids. Employed, funny, and really handsome. Do you mind if I give him your information?"

I hadn't had a date in months. I paused for a second and looked up.

Really? Is that all it took?

It's not like any date can solve all my problems, but it doesn't hurt to get back up on the horse.

Thank you, universe, for showing me the next steps for my highest good and the highest good of all involved.

(And you too, Jesus.)

❖ ❖ ❖

Chapter Nine
Some Things Can't
be Fixed with a Bag of Ice

Facebook Status:

Heard on Michigan Avenue: "What should we do for our anniversary?" a woman asked the man next to her. "Why do you care? We always end up doing what *you* want to do anyway," he said.

⚜ ⚜ ⚜

I make it a point to try to avoid passing my old house whenever possible. Sometimes it is unavoidable, but if I can go another way I do. If Britt and I happen to drive by together, sometimes he will sigh. At first I thought it was in my imagination, but after a while I would hear him say, "I miss the old house, Mom."

"Me too, honey."

It's not like I miss the tax bill or the water bill or what a pain in the ass it was to clean. I miss the hope that it represented. (And my master bedroom.)

Driving past it one day (by accident?) I noticed a truck in the driveway. They were painting the garage door and the shutters a terrible puke brown.

What are they doing to my house?

I remembered how tedious a task it was trying to match that garage door paint to the trim. It took me three trips back to the paint store to get it right. And now they were defacing it with a color that looked like my dog Max had thrown up everywhere.

Let it go, Jen.

The vibration of my phone snapped me back to reality. I looked down and saw a text that was three paragraphs long.

Doesn't anyone use the phone to call people anymore?!!

At the stoplight, I saw that it was a text from my friend Ingrid, asking once again if she could set me up with her friend.

"Can I give him your cell number? His name is Nick. He's so awesome," she wrote.

If he's so awesome, why is he single? Wait a minute – I'm awesome and I'm single. Scratch that.

"Let's start with email," I responded.

Within two hours I had a lovely, heartfelt email from a divorced father of three who wanted to take me to dinner.

I've been on dates with guys who have one kid, maybe two. But when it gets to three or four I start to panic. (It's hard enough raising one; I can't imagine being in charge of a team.)

Leading up to the date, Nick showed his humorous and playful side in emails. It's hard to find someone who can keep up with my sense of humor and Nick was right there with me. Regardless of that fact

136

that he had three children, I was getting more and more excited for our impending dinner.

The night of the date I arrived a bit early to the restaurant and grabbed a seat at the bar. He showed up right on time. As he walked toward me, it felt as though he were moving in slow motion. He was tall, dark and handsome.

Wow!

I couldn't imagine a better candidate – that is – until he opened his mouth.

"So! How are you?" He said, hitting my shoulder with a limp wrist like my best gay friend from college. "Oh my God this place is precioussssssss!"

*You have **got** to be kidding me.*

I've seen married men who have flair. Some straight guys are very metro-sexual and put my wardrobe to shame. But this man was so effeminate, he made Nathan Lane in *The Birdcage* seem butch.

"Let's sit down," I said, my hopes quickly deflating.

I opened my heart up for this, Jesus?

The conversation was plentiful and I did enjoy Nick's personality. But after references to the Neil Diamond songs on his I-Pod and his love for musicals, I was done. I had no desire to take on a relationship with a guy who I suspected was in denial about his sexuality.

He insisted on walking me to my car, but I lied and said I had to head back to work to pick up some books. I really just wanted to be alone. As we said goodbye, he asked about meeting again. I half-heartedly agreed but felt it would never happen.

I started walking and let out a huge sigh. I'd hoped things would be easier after my Match.com debacle, but dating was just as bad the second time around.

This sucks.

The streets were crowded and I tried to flag down a cab. I kept losing out to younger people wearing less clothing.

I decided to keep walking, despite the fact that I had about a mile to go. The weather was nice and my shoes were comfortable so I figured I'd walk the whole way to get some fresh air.

Weekends without your kid – minus a relationship – are painful. So much so, I was having these pangs of wondering, "If my ex isn't happy, and I'm not happy, perhaps we could be unhappy together?"

But we already lived that reality during the last year of our marriage.

I'd heard the saying "what you resist persists" many times from several different spiritual leaders. The basic gist of this is: if you keep trying to push something away it will push back with gusto. If you're afraid of losing money, then people will rip you off. If you worry that a guy will cheat on you, he most likely will cheat on you. I had become pretty resentful of people in love; so it seemed that everywhere I turned I saw happy couples. They were showing up in droves.

What if my ex is in love?

The thought of another woman co-parenting my child was too hard for me to wrap my head around.

I looked up to see if hailing a cab was a possibility, but there wasn't a taxi glow in sight. Before I put my head down to continue my crabby stomp to the parking garage, something in front of me looked familiar. I saw the backside of a couple holding hands. Looking closer, I recognized the man's gate. I'd seen that walk a million times. I studied his jeans and his boots to confirm what I feared to be true: That man was my ex. And he was on a date.

Fuck!

I had "resisted" (or manifested) my worst nightmare. (Actually, worse would have been if he and his date had been sitting at the table next to me when I was with a gay man, but this was still pretty bad.)

I tried to fall back and walk slowly so I wouldn't get too close and be detected. Then I realized I wanted to know what they were saying, so I sped back up again. I eventually settled somewhere in the middle. I put my phone up to my ear pretending like I was having a conversation; that way, if they did turn around, I wouldn't look like I was trying to eavesdrop.

They were being really polite to each other, talking a lot and saying things like "really? You did that too?" It definitely seemed to be the "discovery stage" of their relationship.

I wonder how they met?

The street was too loud for me to hear anything specific other than their laughs. They did this a lot and with each new laugh, it felt like a dagger in my heart. Especially hearing his laugh. Part of what I fell in love with was his sense of humor and his laugh.

During one particular moment of amusement, she leaned into him and he put his arm around her.

I wanted to crawl into the gutter and die.

That used to be my shoulder to lean on.

I tried to study her physique. She was wearing a dress and sandals with a slight heel. Her hair was brown, (although I detected a hint of blonde on the ends) and her body was petite. I started making up careers for her in my head. First she was a yoga instructor. Then she was a waitress. I settled on her being the vice president of a successful P.R. firm.

I wonder if she has kids.

After about three blocks (which felt like three miles) they turned left. I sat there for a minute and watched them continue as I pretended to look for something in my purse. Keeping my eyes on them felt like a form of self-inflicted abuse.

He gets funny and pretty and I get the effeminate heterosexual.

At that moment, my phone vibrated. I looked down and saw a text.

"How was your day?"

My heart sunk with a sense of longing as I wrote back.

"Not bad, you?"

The man on the other end of the text lived on the East Coast. I'd met him during a girl's trip a couple years before. He's handsome, funny, and has two kids of his own. He reads my work and gives me insights into my life that I respect and admire. The only hiccup to this fabulous dynamic, however, is the fact that he's "separated" and not divorced. While this wouldn't be so bad if he was making progress on his divorce, the dial hasn't moved on that status in the time that I've known him. I'm starting to think being "separated" is a convenient term for "no longer sleeping with the wife."

I've told a couple friends about this far-away crush and they both tell me the same thing – putting any energy into someone who lives far away and who is still married is a waste of time.

It's nice to have someone to talk to, though ...

"It's looking like I'll be in Chicago the 12th and 13th," he wrote.

I finally arrived at the parking garage and got into my car. I sat in the driver's seat for a minute, my phone in hand, torn on how to respond.

My logical mind knew that spending time with this person wasn't the right thing to do. But my lonely heart was anxious for some company.

"Sounds good," I wrote.

⚜ ⚜ ⚜

A couple weeks later, I received an email from some co-workers about the company softball league.

"Who's in? No offense to the guys, but we need females."

I've always been athletic. As a kid I took pride in the fact that I batted clean-up and was the only girl on our junior baseball team.

"I'm in," I wrote. I knew none of the people taking part but figured this was a good way to make new friends.

The first game was June 20th.

Shit.

Not only had June 20th been my wedding anniversary, it was also the birthday of my former mother-in- law and the day of my Dad's funeral. He died on Father's Day in 2001.

I hate June 20th.

"Get your toys together," I said to Britt, as he was packing up his things to go to his Dad's for a few days.

"Fine," he said in protest. My son had an elaborate set up of trucks and cars that he had to deconstruct and then reconstruct with each switch of custody. It broke my heart to see him pack his bags.

I did this. We did this to you. I'm so sorry.

"Mom, why doesn't Dad just sleep here?" Britt asked, reluctantly putting his cars into his backpack.

His father and I had been getting along so well, Britt didn't under-stand why we weren't a family anymore. When I was a kid, I never wanted my parents to be in the same state. Now Britt was facing the opposite problem.

"Well honey, when Daddy and I were living together, we didn't get along so well," I tried to explain. "But things are different now that we don't live together and we are really good friends."

Britt still looked sad as he grabbed his "binkers" (a small blanket that is so gross it's beyond description) and put it in his bag. When his dad arrived to get him we exchanged our usual pleasantries.

I wonder if he remembers that today was our anniversary.

"I'm gonna miss you, Mom," Britt said, grabbing my mid-section for a hug.

"I'm gonna miss you so much too, honey," I said, kissing him goodbye.

I watched them get into the car and tried to smile and wave. He was holding back tears, and so was I. Even though this had been our routine for over a year, the process still stung like a fresh wound.

I thought about Britt's question.

Did we make a mistake?

In my logical mind, I knew that getting divorced had to happen for us to get to this point of co-parenting and communicating. Had we stayed a couple, our resentment would have taken center stage. Britt was better off this way.

Right?

But on a day that would have been my wedding anniversary, it took a lot of self-control and positive thinking to avoid feeling sorry for myself.

⚜ ⚜ ⚜

That night, I got to the softball game ready to play. The group welcomed me with open arms but I started to feel nervous.

"I haven't played in a few years," I said. "The last time I did this, I broke my middle finger," I added, showing them the now permanent bend on my right hand.

"That's softball in Chicago," one man said, holding up his pinky with a strange shape that could only come from a broken bone.

As we started things off, I was put in short-right field – the typical assigned position for women.

Before I had time to complain a left-handed batter got up to the plate and hit a line drive right for my head. I put both hands up in the hope of either catching the ball or slowing it down. When I made contact I felt a sting in one of my left fingers. While I didn't catch the ball, I did stop a home run; but I felt like a failure for not making the out.

Why didn't you catch that ball?

"Are you OK? That was quite a line drive," the guy playing second base said.

"I'm fine," I said, shaking my tingling hand.

I looked down and felt a throbbing on my left ring finger.

"Does anyone have some tape?" I asked when we came in from the outfield. I thought I'd sprained the finger, and the best thing to do was just to ice it right away.

After taping two of my fingers together I stuck my left hand in the beer cooler and let the ice soothe the pain.

"How's the finger?" the guy making the lineup asked.

"Fine," I said, still wincing.

I played the rest of the game with a taped hand, but could feel the pain increasing by the moment.

"You coming out for a beer, Jen?" one of the women asked after the game.

"I have to get home to my son," I lied.

All I wanted to do was get home and ice my swollen finger. I stopped by Walgreens on the way to get a splint and some tape. My left ring finger was now completely purple, and as I looked at the colors still forming on my skin, it hit me:

You broke your wedding ring finger on what would have been your wedding anniversary.

This took "what you resist, persists" to a whole new level.

I iced the finger all night, still hoping that deep down it was merely a sprain. I'd see how it felt the next day before deciding if I wanted to get it looked at by a specialist.

When I woke up, the finger was still purple and swollen.

Bzzzzzzzzzz.

My phone alarm was going off, reminding me that I had my annual appointment with my gynecologist in an hour.

Creating small talk when a doctor sticks metal objects into your vagina can be quite awkward. (At least this time around I had a story to jump-start the conversation).

"So I was playing softball yesterday on what would have been my 14th wedding anniversary, and I took a ball to the hand and jammed my wedding ring finger," I said, my doctor's head still under the paper sheet as he inspected my uterus.

"Are you sure you didn't break it?" he asked, "You're going to feel a little pressure here, so sorry."

"I think it's just sprained, but I'm not sure," I said, my voice going up an octave.

When he finished that portion of the exam, he began to check my breasts for lumps. The sight of my splinted hand resting on my stomach made him gasp.

"I know that fingers aren't my area of expertise, Jen, but this finger is not sprained. It's definitely broken," he said.

Definitely broken?

The man who delivered my child was holding my wedding ring finger and telling me in the most gentle but simple terms, "it's broken."

The marriage is broken too.

Some things can't be fixed with wishful thinking and a bag of ice. Things break. Now it was up to me to accept it.

⚜ ⚜ ⚜

The next day, I called my therapist whom I hadn't spoken to in months and asked for a session.

When I went in, I told her all about my broken finger and what Britt had said, and that my ex and I were getting along.

"Did you come here for a refresher course on why you got divorced?" she asked.

"I guess I did," I said. "Is that normal?"

"Very normal," she said. "Now that you aren't living together you are seeing the best in each other. The time that was hardest for you two was when Britt went to bed and before Britt got up. When your child wasn't there to be the buffer."

I already knew everything she was telling me but I needed to hear it again.

"This is why people have more than one kid," I said. "Because they forget how painful childbirth is. It's kind of like that. I have forgotten how difficult things became because I'm only seeing the good stuff."

"Exactly," she said.

She took a minute to write a few things down.

"So how's dating going?" she continued.

"Pretty disappointing," I said. "I was at a dinner the other night with a guy and I asked him, 'how long have you been divorced?' and he said, 'oh I'm not divorced. I'm still living with my wife and daughter.' I said, 'so how does this work? Do I drop you off in the alley, then you flicker the lights so I know you're OK?'"

"It will get better," my therapist said. "You're just starting out. You'll see."

Thank you, universe for helping things to get better. Please. I need things to get better. Soon.

⚜ ⚜ ⚜

Chapter Ten
Tale of Two Theories

Facebook Status:

"Don't try and win over the haters; you are not a jackass whisperer."
-Brene Brown

⚜ ⚜ ⚜

The first time I met Caroline Myss was after her book Sacred Contracts had just been released. I was a reporter for CBS and pitching a story on a woman who claims to be a "medical intuitive" was a hard sell.

In the years that followed we stayed in touch and became friends. One afternoon she invited me over for tea. I'd just missed her birthday celebration and had finished reading her latest book, "Archetypes. Who Are You?"

On the way to her home I pulled over to check my directions. As I eased back into traffic a car ran a stop sign and missed my driver's side by what seemed to be less than a centimeter.

OH MY GOD!!

I was so startled by how close the car came to slamming into my door that I started shaking.

I wondered about the significance of my near-miss as I cautiously drove the rest of the way to Caroline's. Perhaps I needed to be more aware? Maybe I needed to remember how precious life really is.

Or maybe some asshole just ran a stop sign!

Within minutes my phone rang. It was my handyman who was fixing the stairs in my house,.

"We should be all set," he said.

"Until something else goes wrong," I groaned.

My house was ancient, leaving a list of to-do's that never seemed to end. I put down my phone as I pulled up to Caroline's gorgeous Victorian Queen Anne home.

*I want **her** house.*

While Caroline's house also had age, it was restored and painted like a shining gem. I sat for a minute and tried not to be overwhelmed with house envy.

She's a best-selling author, Jen. She worked hard for this. Be grateful for what you have.

Before getting out of the car I reached for a small gift I had in the back seat.

I walked up to Caroline's front door and rang the bell. Her living room looked like a movie set, with exquisite decorating and antiques in every room.

"Great to see you," she said, hugging me at the door.

I walked through the entryway and saw a pile of presents sitting on a bench. From stained glass, to hand made ornaments, she had quite a stash. I looked down at the small bag in my hands with one of my favorite aromatherapy candles I'd planned to give to Caroline as a belated birthday gift.

This present sucks.

Perfectly restored dark wood complemented every room, top to bottom. We made our way to her kitchen as Caroline took the bag from my hands.

"This is very kind, thank you!" she said.

"I love this kitchen."

"I designed it. Head to toe."

My kitchen is the size of a small closet. Every time I cook dinner, I long to be in a home with real countertops.

"It's just gorgeous," I said.

You will have a normal-sized kitchen again, Jen. Someday.

Our conversation began over her birthday festivities. There was a gathering of friends and family, and one of our mutual friends had forgotten to forward the e-vite my way.

"I really feel like I've become fine wine," she said. "Like all the crushing and all the fermenting is over. I just feel like I'm a bottle of fine wine. It's a great feeling."

My phone buzzed. I looked down and saw a text from my ex.

"Let me turn this off," I said, reading the note. "It's my ex texting about our schedule for next week."

"How's that going?" Caroline asked.

"Pretty well actually," I said. "We've gotten to a place where we are putting Britt first. It's very healthy. But I still miss things we did together. Especially around the holidays or our anniversary. I tend to get nostalgic."

"Your ex is an oak. He may not be the biggest oak in the yard, but he's an oak. You can call from anyplace anywhere and he'd be there," she said. "What's going on with the other guy?"

Caroline knew I had a crush on a man who didn't live in Chicago.

"He's supposed to come to town in a few weeks," I said.

"Is he still married?" She asked.

"Yep," I said.

Caroline sipped her tea and looked me right in the eye.

"Do you want me to flush your head in the toilet now or should I wait to do it just before you leave?"

I tried to laugh, but could tell Caroline was kind of not kidding.

"Look, you don't need to be in contact with that man," she said. "But your ex – he's a solid mark."

A solid mark..

"What are you going to do if he finds somebody else?" she asked.

"It will be very hard but that's part of getting divorced," I said.

"And when you find somebody else?" she asked.

"I'm open to it," I said. "But I'm also really getting to the point where I think I'll be OK if I don't have another partner."

Caroline then went on to explain how she had a great love of her life but because of certain circumstances, they couldn't be together. He passed away, but she still feels a strong connection to him in her heart.

"I think it's a mythology – that romantic myth that the person you love the most is the person you always end up with," she said. "That's that child's romantic myth. Love is such a non-negotiating force. Politics and money have a lot more to do with what makes the world go 'round than love. Love has never had an influence on what makes the world go 'round. It has never governed the Vatican."

"I keep watching people who trade problems for problems when the bloom falls off the rose; but after that initial rush wears off, I believe that's when the real relationship starts," I said.

"Part of it is because romantic love is an ideal. The honeymoon period is the love that happens in the fog before you really see the person. If there's a thread of real love in there, then you hold onto that and that's what you use to start weaving the cloth of your life together. We need to love the person's character; his values, his relationships with his own heart; his own soul, his own being; how this person sees life. It's not just about whether this person can support me. It's the quality of who this person is. Then you stand a chance of actually weaving a life cloth together."

My ex and I did have a deep love that produced an incredible child. I started to wonder if I could ever give myself to someone completely the way I did when I got married.

"Do you think we can have more than one great love in our life?" I asked.

"I think the idea that there's one special love applies to some people. I do. But it's not a rule that applies to everybody. Some people do have one special love in their life and that's it. It's not the same for everybody. It's just like some people are going to have kids and some aren't. You can't make a rule about it. It's all relative. Some people require a certain partner and that's all there is to it. They require THAT partner. With other people, maybe they don't love that deeply yet. They're not loving at the soul level but still loving at the ego level, so they're finding relationships that can reflect it – you make me look good. You make me feel good. So the relationship is all about how the other person serves them instead of, 'How can I be your companion in this life? Let me witness your life and you witness mine.'"

"When we first met you told me about how women need to put themselves first every once in awhile, and that it was not considered selfish but rather self-first, like putting your oxygen mask on before helping your small child when the plane goes down," I said. "Do you still believe we should do a little something for ourselves to be better spouses, employees, moms, or even friends?"

"I think I'd be cautious about saying that today because I think we have become such a narcissistic society that the wisdom of that has also given people permission to become very selfish again. It's come full circle. I think now we've gotten where it's really a complex answer, Jen, because we've created a hybrid spirituality in which we have defined the exploration of the self as a spiritual path, and it's not. It's not. Going into therapy and self-indulgence and massage and yoga – this isn't a spiritual path. What's that got to do with a spiritual path? A spiritual path is the pursuit of truth. It's the pursuit of going deeply into self-knowledge and examining questions like … what is my relationship to greed? How much authority does the fear of being humiliated have over me and how much does that fear cause me to harm others? What bargains have I made with darkness? Do I consciously make dark decisions that I know others will pay for? Do I consciously make a bargain with darkness, and am I strong enough to break that bargain? That's a spiritual path. This other stuff about 'look who hurt me,' that's self- indulgent narcissism. So when I talk about putting the mask on first, what I would say today is that you have to be a really wise person to be able to say that. You have to really know what you're talking about."

"Give me an example of what you would consider an appropriate use of putting your mask on first," I asked.

"So, I recently had a number of wonderful people invited to a significant event, and there was a person that is one of those people who comes in and out of my life. I knew that given who this individual was, she would disrupt the entire alchemy of this event. That's the kind of energy this person has. A number of people have bad feelings about this person and in this small room, people would avoid her. It would take clusters to avoid her. She called and said, 'what are you doing?' and I said, 'this event is being thrown' and I could tell she wanted me to just say, 'oh, why don't you come?' Now putting your oxygen mask on first: what does taking care of yourself actually mean? It means making a decision that's not going to feel good. It's acting against my normal compassionate nature. To actually know that this is going to hurt this person – but it would hurt me more to give in. And I could not give in. As soon as I cut the phone call off, I felt something right happen. Something went right in the universe for me. That was putting my mask on first. I followed truth. Maybe putting my mask on is so that I have enough oxygen to carry your load in the world on my back for one more day because that's what's being asked here. Maybe I need more oxygen so you can sleep through the afternoon because you are so exhausted and I'm not. We have to redefine what 'put your mask on first' means."

"I was at a fundraiser last night and I was talking to this woman who lost everything when her husband left her, but she told me she still has a vision board and plays the lottery," I said. "What do you think of people who have their affirmations and put pictures of things they hope will happen or things they want in their life on vision boards?"

"I think it's nonsense. Unmitigated consummate nonsense. I can't tell you how appalling I think it is. There's a passivity that goes along with this psyche that so many people have in today's spiritual movement. This whole idea that, 'if I scream enough or moan enough or pout enough, that someone will come to the rescue and I will not have to do that work myself.' People want someone else to do the work for them. Do you know where my angst comes from? All you are doing is trying to control and get what you want. And that's the thing that I can't tolerate. That's the thing that I find so offensive. Since when do you know what's best for you? Everything that's screwed up about your life, that's what you had a hand in. Everything that was beautiful, you didn't see it coming."

Caroline got up to add more hot water to her mug.

"Would you like a homemade chocolate chip cookie?" She asked, showing me a container of what looked to be delicious home baked goods.

"Yes please," I said.

I looked out the window and saw a cardinal chirping on the tree.

Hi Dad.

"Do you believe people on the other side can send signs?" I asked.

Caroline brought back a plate with some cookies and sat back down at the table.

"I think that we have such a longing to be in touch with people on the other side – I mean I would love to think that Donald, the love of my life, sends me signs. I have to admit that I look for them from him and sometimes I think I even can feel him a little bit. I would have to say that maybe I have. Sometimes I've actually thought 'oh my gosh, you're here,' and the reason I think it was that is because it came out of the blue. I was thinking of something else and it just came – like that. (she snaps her fingers.) In the past when he was alive, I would get that kind of flash – I would – and within an hour I'd get an email from him."

"Do you pray?" I asked.

"Oh yeah. I have a very active prayerful life, and it includes praying for others too – it isn't about me."

"Do you think enough people realize the joy in praying for others?" I asked.

"No, not at all. I know that people don't understand prayer. They don't get what prayer is and why it's powerful. I'm not criticizing them for that because it's like talking to yourself, and we wonder, 'who's out there? Who's listening?' The follow-up word to prayer is *faith* and you have to have faith. But faith in what? You don't see anything changing, or what you do see happening looks even worse than what you were praying for; and you picture the people suffering in Iran and Iraq and Afghanistan and endless war zones and think if they're praying for peace I would've given it up five years ago. So how are their prayers being answered? So prayer is a very mysterious force.

"But as I try to explain to people – and it took me a while to grasp this – prayers can't undo choices we've made. They can't interfere with cycles we've set into motion. For example, we have set into motion several cycles of poison in the environment that are going to have to play out and the praying and praying and praying is not going to undo the cycles of poison. It may cause draughts for 200 years in certain areas. You can pray all you want for rain but it's not going to happen. Now what it *does* do is put the light on so you can see, 'we can't do this again. Help me find a different way. Oh my God. What have I done? Help me find a different way.' And a different way is given."

A different way is given...

⚜ ⚜ ⚜

When I was driving home, a car cut me off on the highway. I looked at the license plate and saw the word "DANIMAL" staring back at me.

I hate vanity plates!

I got home and parked my car in the garage. I tried to close the door and the alignment was slightly off so it wouldn't go all the way down. I wondered about the significance of having my "alignment off" as I kicked the concrete.

It's always something.

As I was walking past my yard to the front door, I noticed a white car stop in front of my house. The man in the passenger's seat was taking a picture of my home with his smartphone.

What the fuck?

"Can I help you?" I asked in a very accusatory tone.

"Oh, I'm sorry," the young man said who was taking the picture. "My grandfather grew up in this house and so we wanted to take a picture."

As I walked closer, I saw that the man who was driving the car looked like an older version of the young man taking the picture. I had a father-son team clicking photos of my house.

"Your grandfather grew up in this house?" I asked.

"Yes," the man driving said. "My father. He loved it here."

He loved my itty-bitty house?

"Is he still with us?" I asked.

"Yep," the son said. "I'm going to email him this picture right now."

"We didn't mean to bother you," the father said.

"No problem," I said. "Tell him that the boiler gives me a little trouble, but otherwise this is a good spot."

This is a good spot, Jen.

"We will," the father said with a laugh. "This is really a great neighborhood."

"Thanks."

They drove away and I took a deep breath and smiled.

I had been putting down my house for months – both internally and to anyone who would listen. I never thought to consider that somewhere, someone not only liked my house but liked it enough to want to see if it was still OK. That somewhere, someone would look at a picture of my mini house and feel nostalgic – maybe even be filled with happy memories of birthday parties or family dinners.

I decided it was time to change the movie in my mind about my house.

You have a beautiful, warm, cozy home, Jen. You are lucky to have a roof over your head. Your glass is half full, not half empty. You are blessed. And life is good.

⚜ ⚜ ⚜

A few days later, there was an email waiting for me from my friend Therese Rowley.

"Hey Jen, do you want to go to Brazil? I want to go see John of God," she wrote.

I'd heard about healer John of God from The Oprah Winfrey Show (before OWN) and from Therese telling me about her visit to see him in Brazil back in the 90's. I was curious to go, but Brazil was really far away.

"I don't know if I can afford to go to Brazil right now," I wrote back. "But let's look into it."

Within minutes, I received an email from someone pitching an interview with a healer by the name of Gail Thackray.

"She works extensively with healer John of God," the pitch said. "Would you be interested in hearing about her work with John of God for your next book?"

Shortly after that email someone at the office also brought up John of God, and how Wayne Dyer claims John of God healed his leukemia.

When I hear about something for the first time it's like a tap on the shoulder. If it comes up again within a short period of time I consider that to be a shove on the side. But three times in 24 hours is the universe's way of hitting me over the head with an anvil.

OK, I get it! I guess I'm supposed to meet John of God.

I arranged to get together with Gail in her hotel lobby for a conversation. I knew she was attractive by her photo, but this blonde-haired blue-eyed bombshell was even more beautiful in person.

"Hello," she said, greeting me with a hug. "So nice to meet you."

We sat down and started to chat. She then explained to me how her life completely changed when out of nowhere, she woke up to discover she had the ability to see dead people.

"I was completely normal – I had three kids, I had businesses, and then the next day I could see spirits," she said. "It was really wild."

Huh?!

"How long ago was this?" I asked.

"This was just when I turned forty, so not that long ago."

"Did something trigger this?"

"My mom and I went to a weekend retreat and it was called 'How to Become a Medium.' I didn't really think anything of it, you know. We had to do these exercises that were supposed to help us bring in a person, and so I said 'I see a man and his name is Grand Pierre

160

Marce; he's talking in French and he is showing me a picture of himself. He was supposed to take over a scaffolding company from his dad and he didn't. He became a pilot.' I knew how he died and I asked, 'is any of that right?' Then this man jumped up and said, yes, that was his name! And he was freaking out and I was totally freaking out because I have no idea how I could do that! I just felt like I'd made it up!"

"Grand Pierre Marce wasn't exactly an average name like John Smith," I said.

"Yes, but that was the name of this man's dead relative and I'd never heard it before. So I went home that night and the spirits wouldn't stop coming in. It was awful. They were telling me, 'you tell my daughter this,' and they were all lined up waiting for me to deliver messages."

"Kind of like in that movie 'Ghost Town' with Greg Kinnear and Ricky Gervais, where Gervais plays the dentist who dies during surgery and has a near-death experience, and when he comes out of it, these spirits keep hounding him to send messages to their loved ones who are still alive," I said.

"Exactly! So I go back the next day to the people who had the retreat and said, 'this is great, but how do I turn this off? I can't function.'"

I tried to imagine the beginning of that conversation.

"Um, hi, so I have these dead people in my living room. Can I please have a refund?"

"I really had to learn how to turn it on and off," she said. "Now I have it figured out, but it was tricky."

161

"Had you ever taken any psychic classes before that retreat?" I asked.

"I had taken Reiki about a month before, and I didn't feel anything. But now I do healings and help people and it's completely changed my life."

"So what's your process?" I asked. "How do you tap into the other side?"

"I honestly think it's all the same," she said. "I know some people say you have to do certain things and have a certain ceremony, but I think it doesn't matter how you get there. I think once you decide to open up, you then connect to the other side. I think we're all mediums. We can all do this. We can all get messages from loved ones. We can all have energy channeled to us and heal people; but I think with our judgments and fears, we mentally block it out."

"What did your family think when this change happened to you?" I asked.

"When this all started happening, my husband thought I was completely nuts – I mean, he believed me because I was telling him things he couldn't possibly know, but he was totally freaked out."

"Are you still married?"

"No," she said. "And that was definitely why. It really changed my life, but I think for the better and he didn't believe in it."

"Tell me about John of God," I asked.

"When you meet him, everything changes," she said. "It's wonderful. I've witnessed incredible healings and surgeries that John of God has done. When you go to someone like John of God the healing is all done through God or a higher being, and John of God is like the go-between. He is doing God's work. Most people aren't able to tap into that power directly. John of God can. People who go to him are getting healed, not just physically, but emotionally. I think all of our issues – whether they're financial, emotional or health issues – can be healed. It's stuff that has collected over time. When you go for a spiritual healing, you're working to heal what caused the illness. So if you have a cancerous tumor and you go and get that removed, then you go back to life; but if you don't deal with what caused it or it will come back."

I wonder if he can heal my heart?

"So people have to do some work on themselves too," I said. "It's not just John of God waving his hand and healing everything permanently."

"Yes. Even today, when I work on people, I've found with spiritual healings that I do now, I would fix somebody and it would last for a while, and then they would come back with the same problem. I tell people I don't want them to keep coming to see me. I want to inform people that they can do it themselves and show them that they can do it."

"What's your mantra?" I asked.

"I don't have a mantra. I just believe that we should trust source. I call it God. Trust that there is an energy out there – source energy – and there is a whole universe there to help us."

Gail looked at me with a slight squint in her eye.

"You're very clarsencient," she said. "You can feel other people's feelings, and I'm surprised at what you do for a living because you pick up stuff from other people."

My whole life I've had issues where I take on other people's angst. I've had to work very hard to keep this in check.

"Also, people at work will come and tell you their problems and you talk to them and they feel better and then you don't realize why you feel drained. It might not kick in for a couple of days. Sometimes you can even get illnesses and you don't know what it is and the doctor can't pinpoint it, and it's stuff you're picking up from other people."

True, and true.

"Sometimes just the news of the day can get me so upset," I said. "I often try to figure out why bad things happen to good people."

"I do believe that everything that comes to us is because we've asked to have this experience," she said. "The good and the bad. But I think we're supposed to get to a point where everything we have is joyful. I don't think we're supposed to be struggling. I really don't think we are here to be punished. We often bring things to us that are not positive. But we can turn that around and decide to say, 'I think I'm done with that lesson.'"

"So when we face the fear and learn the lesson, then we can experience the joy?" I asked.

"Yes," she said.

Gail's theory went against everything Caroline Myss told me:

"All you are doing is trying to control and get what you want. And that's the thing that I can't tolerate. That's the thing that I find so offensive. Since when do you know what's best for you? "

"When things are going wrong and you get depressed, it's not easy to just say, 'OK, I'm going to think positive now and everything will be fine,'" Gail said. "It's difficult. That is the point when a spiritual healer can help. But sometimes you meet people who go to see every healer they can, and they're constantly searching – looking here, looking there. And I'll say to them, 'it's inside you. Stop searching everywhere else. Stop wanting everyone to fix you. You have to fix yourself.' It's not like I have some special gift. You have what I have. I try to explain to people that they have it and I teach them how to open up and feel it themselves."

"So what's one thing that people can do each day that will help them feel connected to source or the energy that you tap into?" I asked.

"Before you get up in the morning, say, 'I put white light protection all around me,' or 'God protect me' or 'Angels protect me' – whatever you believe. And then decide to open yourself up to God or source, whatever you want to call it. When you walk with the intention that you have white light protection all around you, that is a very powerful thing."

I quickly imagined a white ball of super-awesome protection all around me as we continued our conversation.

"What are your thoughts on people who want to manifest things?" I asked. "I'm kind of torn lately between wanting things and putting those wants into my consciousness, or accepting that maybe God knows what's best for my highest good and that might not involve having more stuff."

"It's very positive to want things that make you happy, so if you want a car that you would love to drive, there's nothing wrong with picturing yourself in that car. But if you want it so you can show off to your neighbor, that's the wrong reason for wanting it. That's coming from the ego."

"For some reason, I've always had the belief that if you want to be spiritual, you shouldn't want to be rich either," I said. "Marianne Williamson told me that the belief that we are holy when we are poor comes from the Bible, and that there is nothing holy about waiting in a bread line. Do you agree?"

"Yes!" Gail said. "God wants us to have joy and abundance. "

But Caroline said God knows what's best for us. I'm so confused!

"When I first started doing readings I had a guy who came to me and he said, 'can you tell me what to invest in for the stock market and futures?' " Gail continued. "So I said 'I don't know if I can do that; let me ask,' and my spirit guides said, 'it's not about choosing the right stocks. He has to decide what he wants to do with that money. If it's just about having $100,000 in the bank, that won't really do it; but if it's to put the grandkids through college because it would make him feel really happy, there's good energy around that. When there is pure energy around something, then he will be guided to pick the right stocks.' But you have to deal in for things to happen. If you ask to manifest something, be sure to watch for the signs you get. Maybe somebody calls you up out of nowhere and says, 'hey, let's get together for dinner.' You've gotta play the 'yes' game and watch what happens. Get involved in life. You will meet someone who takes you to the next level. A lot of times guides will open the door and give you opportunities and you sit at home and say, 'I don't really feel like it.' Opportunity isn't just going to drop in your driveway. And it might come in a different form than you expect. You have to be active about it in order to receive it."

It's not going to drop in my driveway? Dammit!

That night I decided to create a vision board of my own. It wouldn't include pictures of houses or headlines about my job aspirations and writing career, but rather images of things that helped me feel happy and peaceful. I secretly wondered if Caroline would scold me as I cut and glued my gorgeous images. From a statue of Buddha to a waterfall in the tropics, every item had a purpose and created a sense of calm within my being.

You gotta deal in for things to happen ...

⚜   ⚜   ⚜

CHAPTER ELEVEN
FEAR IS LIKE A BEACH BALL

Facebook Status:

"Yes, I'd like to place an order.... I'd like the man of my dreams and eternal bliss. For here please."

❧   ❧   ❧

I was sitting at my desk one day and a note came through from a Facebook friend.

"I'm trying to get Anita Moorjani to come to Chicago," she wrote. "I will let you know as things progress."

Anita Moorjani is the woman Wayne Dyer told me about who had 24 cancerous tumors, some the size of lemons. She fell into a coma and was not expected to live. She came back to life and is now fully healed. Her healing remains a mystery to the medical community and her book. "Dying To Be Me" was a New York Times bestseller. I've been fascinated by her story ever since Wayne first brought her to my attention.

After the Facebook message, I went through my notes from my conversation with Wayne. To my complete surprise, he gave me Anita's email address.

Even though she lived in Hong Kong, I decided to send her a note asking if she was interested in coming to Chicago. I also asked if she would be willing to be interviewed for my book.

She said "yes" to both requests.

Holy shit!

We set up a time to Skype a few days later. At 6 a.m., I sat at my desk in my pajamas talking in cyberspace with a woman who had one of the most impressive cancer recoveries ever documented.

"It's so nice to meet you," she said.

Meet ME? I'm not the one who died and lived to tell about it!

"Some people don't get to come back and have this 'ah- ha' as you have," I said. "Do you have moments where you wonder, 'why me?'"

"Yes, I've had a lot of moments when I've wondered 'why me?' I also feel that the ones who didn't come back are very blessed because it was so amazing on the other side, it really was. I feel that the ones who got to stay are not the unfortunate ones."

"I interviewed Dr. Mary Neal who also died and wrote about it in the book, 'Heaven and Back,' and I asked her why do bad things happen to good people. She said she doesn't believe there are bad things. What is ... just is. Do you agree with that?" I asked.

"I absolutely agree with that. I tell people that everything that happens to us is a gift, even my cancer was a gift; and in hindsight when we look back we can see that everything that was an obstacle is a gift. When people say to me the cancer nearly killed me, I say, 'no, the cancer saved my life.' I was already killing myself with all of my fears before I had cancer. I do truly feel in the end everything is a gift, and if it doesn't feel like a gift at the time it means we haven't reached the end yet."

"How long ago did you go into the coma?" I asked.

"It's coming up on seven years," she said.

"Is your memory just as strong as when it happened to you?"

"It is just as strong. The reason why is because when I was in that state, it felt like *that* state was the awake state. And *this* is the dream state. People have asked me, 'how can you be sure that wasn't a dream?' and I say I'm positive because when we have a dream, over time the dream fades and this hasn't faded. I like to use the analogy that if you imagine you were blind, that you were born blind and you have never been able to see in your life, you don't know what colors are, what perspective is, what distance really means. Then imagine one day you suddenly have sight. And maybe you have sight for 24 hours or 48 hours. And suddenly you have this incredible clarity, and you see colors and distance. I was in the coma for 30 hours – and then if that sight is gone again, even though it's gone, if you go back to being blind, you cannot undo that knowledge which you have been given, which now changes your perspective on how the whole world looks. It changes how you see the world. That never leaves you and that's kind of how it feels."

"I've recently interviewed two people with different perspectives on abundance," I said. "I'm torn inside between thinking that we can have everything we desire and then thinking, well, God has a plan and maybe his plan is for some suffering to happen so I can appreciate what comes later. How do you feel about manifesting?"

"I have a very different way of manifesting," she said. "I don't go through the vision board or the power of intention or anything ...

because, here's what I believe: it's human nature to have desires. You have dreams, and that's fine, it's part of being human and you can't suppress them. The more you suppress them the more you are not allowing yourself to be who you are. But in order to attract what is truly yours, you only have to love yourself and allow yourself to be who you truly are. The more you love yourself, the more you will allow those things that you desire to find you. The more you don't like yourself or criticize and judge yourself or beat yourself up – the more you will suppress yourself and make yourself small. You will be pushing away your dreams and desires and everything that is truly yours. Just love yourself unconditionally and your external world will reflect what you feel inside."

There's that damn 'loving yourself' piece again ...I can't get away from this.

"What advice would you give people who let fear seep in?"

"Don't judge the fear, because the more we judge it the more it will push back," she said. "It's like a beach ball: when you are trying to push it under the water, the more it pushes back. So the first thing you have to do is accept the fears. Once you accept them and embrace them, then the next thing you have to do is to find what brings you joy in life and do what brings you joy. Ask yourself, 'if this fear wasn't here, what would I do?' And listen for that answer, and then go and do it. Do what brings you joy. Because the thing about life is there's no room for joy and fear to exist simultaneously. It's always one or the other. And when you get into the habit of waking up everyday and saying, 'what do I do that brings me joy?' what you'll find is there's less and less fear."

"I love that analogy of the beach ball," I said. "It's so true. What you resist persists."

171

"That's right. Don't push the fear out because it will push back," she said. "Reach for something else so you are replacing it, you're not pushing the fear out, you're actually going for something else. I tell people that we spend so much time focusing on cancer awareness campaigns, if we put as much time focusing on **wellness** campaigns and **health** campaigns, and spent money on that, that's what we would be creating instead of illness and cancer. It's not about pushing something away; it's about growing something that you want instead."

Growing something that you want instead.

"How can we help parents and kids with this?" I asked.

"I think we do our kids a disservice when we tell them that they have to do this or they have to do that. When they're not allowed to find their own strengths and their own talents, they're trying to measure up to what we want of them and their teachers want or what their peers are doing and they wind up falling short and feeling inadequate. We're creating generations and generations of kids who are competing with each other and trying to outdo each other, and they always end up feeling like they fall short. We need to teach them that they are unique, and they need to find their own strengths and their own talents and whatever their talents are – that they have value. The universe needs all of us. Be as YOU as you can be. And if you stop being you, the universe will be deprived of who you came here to be."

"Having been in the light, what are your beliefs about religion now?" I asked.

"Everybody is gonna die, and it doesn't matter if you are Christian, Muslim, Hindu, Jewish, it doesn't matter. To believe that there is a God of a particular religion that is going to punish for all of eternity anybody who doesn't follow a particular kind of religion is to say you believe this GOD, universal energy, whatever you want to call it, is very cruel. So we've given religion these traits that are actually not true. When we cross over, the love is absolutely unconditional; and if you believe that your chosen religion is unconditionally loving, then you cannot believe that people will be punished for not believing in that religion. Because it's a contradiction."

"Do you believe there's a heaven and hell?" I asked.

"I don't believe there is a hell at all. I believe that in the other realm we awaken. It is purely positive. I believe that some people do experience some darkness before getting into the light. Some people have experienced darkness in their near-death experience, and they believe that it's hell. But I believe that darkness is still their mind being attached to beliefs in this world. I know, I absolutely know, that those who experience darkness have not gone all the way into the light yet, because it's still part of the mind attachment to this world. Once they go beyond that and let go, everybody goes to this same realm, which is unconditionally loving. That is the final place."

Unconditionally loving.

"I was on the Jeff Probst Show a few weeks ago," she continued. "I used the word nirvana instead of heaven because to me, it's just a label and it's the same thing; and I got incredible feedback from that and lovely emails; but I got one email from somebody out of thousands – one email from one woman who said, 'I noticed you said nirvana instead of heaven. I feel very sorry for you that you did not attribute it to our one and only Jesus Christ. What happened to you? I pray for you that when you finally die that you will go to heaven.' This kind of thinking is a cancer! And you know what's interesting? In that interview I said I grew up a Hindu, so I wondered, is she saying that everyone who grew up a Hindu or a Muslim, they're all going to that same place that she's referring to?

It still surprises me in this day and age that people are so judgmental and intolerant."

This kind of thinking is a cancer...

"I did a book talk, and a woman pulled me aside and said she was going to pray for my soul since I was going to hell for the title of my book, 'I'm Spiritual, Dammit!'" I said.

"Wow! We really have our work cut out for us, Jenniffer," Anita said. "Imagine what would happen if they shifted that energy from hate to love. It would be incredible."

⚜　⚜　⚜

A couple days later I was driving with my son and his friend and the friend said,

"Wow! Look at THAT house!"

We were on my old street and he was pointing to my old house.

"Out of all the houses on this block, he picks out mine," I laughed.

It's not yours anymore, Jen.

I thought about the words of Anita:

"It's like a beach ball: when you are trying to push it under the water, the more it pushes back."

"We used to live in that house," I said.

"Really?"

"Yes," I said. "But now we have a different house and we like that one just as much."

I looked in the rear view mirror to see if Britt was OK. He was playing his game and had a smile on his face.

I turned the music up and kept on driving.

"Don't push the fear out because it will push back. Reach for something else..."

⚜   ⚜   ⚜

CHAPTER TWELVE
YOU GOTTA FIX YOURSELF BEFORE
YOU CAN FIX THE WORLD

Facebook Status: Two young men were chatting in line at Starbucks. The one in a suit said to the one who looked like he was wearing pajamas: "Yeah, I'd like to have someone change my diapers, feed me, pay my bills, and decide my schedule too, but the deal is, I'm not a year old anymore, dude! Get off your ass!"

☙ ☙ ☙

Reality shows kind of piss me off because most of them celebrate conflict and thrive on people with low self-esteem. But I can appreciate the sentiment behind a singing show that discovers unknown talents.

One afternoon at work I was scrolling through different singing videos and came across a segment from the show, "Britain's Got Talent" with Simon Cowell.

A beautiful 28-year old "beauty therapist" named Alice Fredenham was telling the camera she didn't tell anyone she was auditioning for the show because "I just thought I'd rather go at it alone and then if I'm not successful I don't have to admit that to anyone."

In the video she walks on the stage with her posture slightly slumped, wearing a simple white sweater and her dark hair pulled back. And then, with a voice like satin, her body relaxes as she delivers a jazzy version of "My Funny Valentine" that knocks the judges' socks off.

"Oh – my – God," Cowell gushes. "This is what I've been waiting for. Your voice is like liquid gold.

You have such an authentically beautiful voice. You look amazing."

At this point, Alice starts balling. It's as if she can't believe her ears.

"You could sing the phonebook," Cowell continues. "I absolutely love you and I love your voice. And I also love the fact that you actually don't even know how good you are."

"Why are you crying, Alice?" another judge asks.

"I just don't think I ever expected this kind of response," she says. "It's like my dream ... and now it's just happened."

I really could relate to Alice because I, too, suffer from low self-esteem. When I was growing up my father had very high standards. He got them from his father who expected the best, yet never dished out a compliment in his life. With my Dad's side of the family you were never praised. (They would praise you to strangers or other people, but never to your face.)

Looking back, I see how damaging this was. I didn't have an internal compass that helped me gauge what I could do well. My mother tried to pick up the slack and tell my brother and me that we could do anything we set our minds to. But I have a theory that people who weren't praised by their fathers spend the rest of their lives trying to get that praise (even if their dad happens to be dead, which was the focus of my first book).

My video screening was suddenly interrupted by a call from the front desk.

"Jenniffer, Sara is in the lobby," the security guard said.

Sara Morrison was a sweet 16-year-old girl who emailed me after she found my book, "I'm Spiritual, Dammit!" as she was wandering through a suburban bookstore.

"The title just spoke to me," she wrote.

After her initial email we'd started a dialogue and talked about everything from her struggles with finding a religion that matched her idea of spirituality to coping with new friends in high school. Each time I spoke with Sara I was amazed at her wisdom. As a teen-ager she had a better sense of self than most adults.

"Hey you," I said, greeting her in the lobby. "My lunch break just started, so let's go sit somewhere and catch up."

"How's the book coming?" she asked.

"It's taking all these twists and turns," I said. "A lot of it is focusing on my ability to love myself no matter what, which is really hard."

"I had struggles with that," she said. "I started with a therapist at age 10."

Sara seemed really grounded, and her parents were happily married. I'd always assumed kids who went to therapy came from broken homes.

"Did you have to shop around for a good one?" I asked.

"No, I got the perfect person right off the bat. But I was lucky. I've talked to so many people about their problems and they say 'I feel so alone' and I will say, 'you should go and talk to a therapist because it could really help you because they really helped me,' and one of the most common responses I get from people is, 'I have one and they're terrible and I hate them,' and I ask, 'why are you still with that person? Go find someone else.'"

"Why did you need a therapist at the age of 10?" I asked.

"For a long time growing up I didn't like myself very much. I felt guilty when I felt happy! I felt like I was a terrible person for having a good life. I felt like people hated me for being happy; so I hated myself because I felt everyone else hated me too."

My heart broke thinking of a girl who thought she was hated for being too happy.

"I'd read a book called, "The Golden Compass" where everyone has these animals who assist them," she said. "It's their soul embodied in a little animal. They're called daemons. So after I read the book I remember thinking 'wouldn't that be cool to have a daemon?' I was about 12 at the time. I decided in an imaginary friend sort of way that I would have one. I developed a very strong connection to mine."

This daemon piece was sounding a bit strange, but I knew a lot of people who had imaginary friends growing up, so I kept listening.

"One day I was sitting in the car and feeling really horrible about myself," she continued. "I had a friend who hated everyone and every-thing. She attempted suicide a couple of times and I was trying to save her. I felt so terrible about everything because nothing I did would help her. I was sitting in the car and my mom was in the store and I just started crying. My daemon had been comforting me a lot, but when I reached for him in the car, he started fading. It was like he was disappearing into thin air. I reached out to him, saying, 'come back!

I love you,' and he said, 'I'm a part of you; I'm your soul; and if you don't love yourself, you can't possibly say that you love me.' I realized that if I didn't try my hardest in that moment to love myself that I was going to lose him forever and I was going to be alone. I didn't think of it as losing myself but that's definitely what it was."

Who has these thoughts at the age of 12?

"So how did you soothe yourself?" I asked.

"I reached as deep into myself as I could and I found this little bit inside of me that was fighting to never, ever, give up hope that I was a good person and the world was a good place, even though there were bad things that happen all the time. I started repeating to myself, 'I love myself, I am strong and I'm beautiful.'"

As she's telling me this I tried to picture my 12-year-old self sitting in a parking lot having a meltdown and soothing myself by saying the words, "I love myself, I am strong and I'm beautiful" to calm myself down.

*I can't even say that shit to my **current** self!*

"It wasn't like from that moment on everything was great and I loved myself," she continued. "It was a long journey. A lot of people had been working with me to get me to love myself – parents, my therapist and friends; but it hadn't worked because I didn't think I was worthy of being loved."

I thought about the Alice Fredenham video from Britain's Got Talent and how she shook her head "no" when Simon Cowell told her she had a voice like an angel.

"Even if the whole world is telling you that you're fabulous, it doesn't matter if you don't believe it inside," I said.

"Right. I thought it was nice of people to say those things, but I felt like they were wasting their time trying to make me feel like a good person."

"How do you feel today?" I asked.

"I don't spend every moment in my life feeling confident," she said. "I don't think anybody does."

No shit.

"But I feel in general like I do love myself. I wish there was more that I could do to spread that idea, because I feel like there's this crisis in my generation. Kids my age don't understand the difference between self-confidence and self-obsession. I think there are so many teenagers who get into a vicious cycle where the only way they know how to love themselves is to be self-obsessed. And then others see that they're self-obsessed and put them down."

I thought about the people in my office who are obsessed with Instagram and Twitter. They can't focus on one task for more than three minutes because they have to post their every move.

"I see this all the time on the Internet," she said. "If someone gets really popular, then people will post anonymous comments like, 'why don't you go and kill yourself?' They'll say really awful things. For a long time I refused to love myself because I was afraid I'd become self-obsessed. I was raised to think self-obsession is so terrible. My parents are Buddhist and that's one of the reasons I decided to leave Buddhism because in Buddhism you're not supposed to focus on yourself."

"Really?" I asked.

"No. You are supposed to help others, which is good too. But I think you should focus on yourself, not in a selfish way, but if you're going to help other people you have to come from a place of peace within yourself. You can't create peace in the world if you're coming from a broken self. You have to fix yourself before you can fix the world. "

❧   ❧   ❧

I went back to my desk after my meeting with Sara and found an email notification from someone requesting to connect on LinkedIn. This "somebody" was a boy from my high school who broke my heart at the age of 15. Shortly before the prom he ended our relationship so he could ask someone else. As a sophomore, I wouldn't have sex or drink beer, and apparently this was a deal breaker for prom night. (If he'd gotten me a little later in my high school career he may have had the time of his life; but I digress.)

That break-up messed with my head until I was out of college – not because he was so incredible but because I was so vulnerable. I looked to boys to fill an emotional hole. High school girls who don't have strong male figures in their lives need a lot of nurturing or their self-esteem will suffer. It bugs me to quote John Mayer, but he was right when he wrote, "Fathers be good to your daughters" because neglected daughters can become bitter mothers and this just repeats a cycle of insecurities. I only saw my Dad on weekends because of my parents' divorce and my Mom and my step dad divorced when I started high school, so for those four critical years, there was no role model around the house.

So when I saw this name on my computer (let's call him Charlie) I had to pause for a second to get my bearings. He taught me to drive a stick-shift. He took me on my first motorcycle ride. He picked me up after school and drove me to the beach in his convertible where we'd roll around on the sand and make out for what felt like hours. He was my Jake Ryan from "Sixteen Candles"; only we didn't have that fairy tale ending with a kiss on the dining room table over the glow of a lit birthday cake.

182

Charlie literally hadn't been on my mind in over 20 years, and seeing that name morphed me into the girl who lived for that moment between gym class and chemistry when I would see him in "H" hall. It reminded me of all the nights I waited by the phone for his call, fighting with my older brother for use of the landline. (This was before cell phones, emails and answering machines).

So back to reality – we exchanged a couple of emails and decided to go to lunch the following week to discuss his new business. He also said he wanted to get my advice on some social media issues.

Before our meeting I tried to do some detective work. Was he married? Divorced? Just feeling nostalgic? I called a friend from high school who kept her pulse on all the gossip to see what I could find out.

"Maybe he's single and after all these years, he can't stop thinking about you?"

"He might be very happily married," I said.

"Or he wants to have a torrid affair," she said.

She made everything sound like the plot of a Lifetime movie.

Not having seen Charlie in decades, my curiosity was off the charts. Would he be fat? Bald? Does he have kids? My brain kept hopping between my teenaged self who cared a LOT and my present-day self who cared maybe a little.

OK, a lot.

As I walked out to the lobby, I saw a man on his phone. He was absolutely stunning. My heart began to race.

Oh my gosh he's so hot!

"Charlie?" I said, looking at a dark-haired man's profile.

The man looked up at me with his phone on his ear, and to my surprise it was a complete stranger.

"Oh I'm so sorry," I said, feeling like an idiot.

I looked to my left, and there he was – a 44-year-old version of "the man who dumped me before prom" as he became known to all my friends in the 80's. He was in need of a haircut and a few pounds heavier, but for the most part, still looked like Charlie.

"I almost hugged the wrong guy," I admitted, giving him an embrace.

As we small talked on our way to the restaurant I got the sense he was slightly nervous. He talked a lot (which is normally my job) as we covered the basics, such as the weather and traffic. Within a couple of minutes we were seated at our destination.

"So ..." I said, looking him straight in the eye. "Tell me about the last 20 years."

As he started to chat I looked at his left hand. No ring.

Interesting.

"Do you have kids?" I asked, hoping this would fill in the blanks.

"Yes. Two daughters and a son," he said.

Still no mention of a wife.

"You?" He asked.

"I have a son who's six," I said. "His father and I are divorced, but we're great friends and live just a mile away from each other."

"That's cool," he said.

That's all you've got??

Before I could find out his marital status the waitress came up to give us the tutorial on the menu. As she left, I couldn't help myself.

"You married?" I asked.

"17 years," he blurts out.

So why the fuck aren't you wearing a ring??

I've had this debate so many times with men who don't wear rings. I feel it's completely false on their part. Either you "wear it loud and wear it proud" or you leave it off because you're not committed to the marriage. Not wearing a ring is false advertising.

"Wow!" I said. "That's awesome."

*And by "awesome" I mean completely **not** awesome.*

I watched him carefully as he looked at the menu. The more I studied him I came to realize he was just a regular guy. I was so pleased that my stomach didn't do flips in his presence. Part of this, I'm sure, is maturity and the other part is that I doubted we had anything in common other than where we got our high school diplomas.

"What's good here?" he asked.

Just as I was picking up my menu I felt this overwhelming sadness for my 15-year-old self. I don't even recognize that girl and yet I know she was a part of me.

You didn't know how to love yourself.

I wanted to shout from the rooftop of every high school to every girl who was rejected by the popular boy,

"Things will get better ladies! And I promise you that there will be a day when you are sitting across from the boy who broke your heart, thinking, 'he's not that great. I mean look at the way his eyebrows hang over his eyes. Doesn't he own a pair of tweezers?'"

"Have you had a chance to look at the menu?" the waitress asked, approaching our table.

"What's your favorite thing?" I asked.

"The chicken thigh kabobs," she said without hesitation.

"Done. Let's get one of those," I said.

"And for you?" she asked Charlie who was still looking down at the menu.

"Do you like mussels?" he asked me.

"Actually, yes. I love mussels."

"Let's do some mussels too," he said to the waitress.

"Great, I'll put those right in," she said, taking our menus.

While I noticed a certain amount of comfort between us, what seemed to be missing was chemistry, which made me relax. I wasn't monitoring my choice of words or worried about putting my elbows on the table. I felt completely neutral.

And as my mother would say, "It's about fucking time!"

The meal progressed, and I quickly learned that while Charlie is married, things aren't all rosy in Charlieville.

Shocker.

He told me that his wife goes out partying until the wee hours of the morning and barely gets his kids to school on time. He said she also acts like a kid around their three children during the day, putting a lot of pressure on Charlie to pick up the parenting slack. I find this to be the case for my friends who got married too young. Once the kids get to be at an age where they no longer need a babysitter, the parents start acting like children.

"She tells me she should be able to do what she wants. And I'm like, 'hello!! We have a family here. You can't just go missing for 12 hours. I don't buy the 'I didn't have my cell phone charger' excuse!"

Go missing? What kind of mother goes missing?!

"I can't believe I'm telling you all this," he said.

"I like to listen, so I don't mind at all," I said.

*Why **is** he telling me all this?*

I then realized the reason I was talking to Charlie in that moment.

He has daughters.

"I want to share something with you, Charlie. When I was dating you in high school I had low self-esteem," I admitted, feeling slightly embarrassed that I was being so honest. "There is nothing more critical than a teenaged daughter having a solid role model. She needs someone who really wants to know about her life. And I don't mean in a controlling way, because as parents we want to control things. But if your daughters are dating, don't harp about the boys' intentions or ask for the gory details. Say something to each daughter like, 'does he have any idea how wonderful and special you are? I sure hope so!' If they don't get that from their dad or some sort of reliable figure when they hit puberty, they will spend the rest of their lives seeking approval from unavailable men. We go with what we know. I can't stress how important it is."

Charlie looked at me intensely. I felt like he wanted to share something but was holding back. And then,

"Our oldest daughter is having some issues," he said. "We're taking her to a therapist right now. She's addicted to her phone and being in touch with her friends."

She is addicted to the approval of others, I'll bet.

"If she doesn't hear from them she gets so depressed. It's like their opinion is the only thing that matters. And if friends don't 'like' things on Facebook or if they 'unfriend' her, it's the end of the world."

"Social media has made us have to work three times as hard to build up our kids' confidence," I said. "If they feel they have a good base and have support at home, they are less likely to have meltdowns when they don't get 'likes' on Facebook or hear from their friends."

"I try to talk to her, but she's so mad at me right now. She slams the door in my face. And I'm always there for her, pumping her up."

"What about her mother?" I asked.

He paused, almost hesitant to answer me.

"She isn't very engaged in what the older kids are up to," he said.

"That's why your daughter is slamming the door in your face," I said. "Anger and rage only come from fear or disappointment. She's afraid or disappointed about something, that's for sure. And she's taking it out on you."

I could see Charlie's mind working hard.

"My wife doesn't want to change and I keep thinking I can change her," he said with a nervous laugh.

And that is the bumper sticker for divorce.

"You can't make someone change," I said. "I wrote a whole column about it. The more you try, the more they fight it. I actually interviewed a woman who told me, 'change only comes from inspiration and not imposition.' You can't force your beliefs onto someone. If you do, they only resent it and they push back even harder."

What you resist persists.

"Just remember, we are teaching our kids what a relationship looks like with our own behavior," I said. "They are like sponges, soaking up every argument or unspoken pet peeve. So if you want her to be in a loving, communicative relationship, that will only happen if you are leading by example."

As we walked out of the restaurant, I got the distinct feeling his marriage was toast.

But I did feel that I was meant to give him that message about his daughters.

⚜ ⚜ ⚜

In the days that followed, Britt had a terrible cold and I was doing everything in my power to avoid getting sick. In the nearly three years I'd been at my job, I'd taken only three sick days. You don't call-in sick for broadcasting or journalism unless you can't speak or write. You work through the hacks and sniffles and suck it up. Of course this stupid mentality means everyone in the office just transfers the cold from one person to the other, but it's just the way it is.

So when I woke up one Monday morning with what felt like a fever, I tried to talk myself out of it.

You can work through it, Jen.

I stood up and immediately felt dizzy. Not only was my nose completely clogged, but my left ear was so plugged up I couldn't hear. My throat felt like it was on fire, and my eyes were crusted shut. I was a terrible combination of hear no evil, see no evil, smell no evil and speak no evil. There was not one sense in my body that was working properly.

What does this mean?!

I hopped in the shower, still trying to convince myself that I could go in to work. Not only was I needed for my writing duties, but on this Monday in particular, I was supposed to be the moderator for an event, as well as get a show ready for a webcast. There were several tasks that needed my attention, and my attention only.

How can you moderate an event when you can't even speak a sentence?

My mom called as I was getting ready for work.

"You sound awful honey," she said. "Stay home today."

"I can't," I said. "We have an event and I'm the moderator."

I blew my nose and a sharp pain shot through my left ear.

You're not superwoman, Jen. It's time to surrender.

"What's the worst thing that can happen if you don't show up?" She asked.

I thought about this for a second. It's not like I would get fired for being sick.

"I don't know who would be able to step in," I said.

"Somebody will step in," she said. "They can figure it out."

The world will continue to spin on its axis even if you don't show up at work.

A CEO consultant once told me that the best thing that can happen in an office is when someone is asked to step in for another to do something they don't normally do. By relinquishing some control, the person who isn't there is giving someone else a chance to take on a new task and show they have what it takes to get things done. This helps every team member stay on their toes so that their skill sets remain fresh and challenged. By letting each employee shine, this makes for a stronger team, he said.

It's time to relinquish some control.

I picked up the phone and called my boss and left a message. Next I called my doctor and made an appointment to get a throat culture.

My diagnosis was as I expected – a sinus infection, ear infection and throat infection. (The eye goop was related to my sinuses.) I was an ear, nose and throat disaster.

I went to the pharmacy to pick up my prescription.

"Can I see your driver's license please?" The pharmacist asked.

"Why do you need my driver's license?" I asked.

"For the Advil Cold and Sinus," she said.

To get a decongestant, I had to sign more paperwork than people who buy guns at Walmart.

Something is very wrong with this country.

When I got home, I plopped onto the couch and turned on the television.

Ricki Lake is back?

I hadn't watched daytime television in years. I felt like a teenager flipping through the channels at lightning speed. Everything was new to me. Ricki was interviewing rapper YK about the loss of his friend and manager Ronnie "Scooby" Chambers who was gunned down while sitting in a parked car in Chicago.

"He kept me protected," YK said about Scooby. "He kept me from the violence and standing on the streets and hanging out and doing bad things. He said I had talent and I could go somewhere with it. And that's what I did. He helped me become somebody."

Holding back tears, Ricki then brought on the national spokesperson for the Rainbow Coalition, Dr. Shawn McMullin.

"In 2012 there were more than 500 murders in Chicago," Ricki said. "In 2013 there have already been 43 murders. What is going on in Chicago?"

No shit!

"Let me say this," McMullin said. "We hear about the numbers and the statistics about what's going on in Chicago....Every year Chicago public schools cannot find 6000 students who drop out between the 8th and 9th grade. Violence doesn't just happen – it's a four-legged stool that stands on certain things. Where there is despair, where there is dilapidated education, where there is access to weapons and where there is grinding poverty you will always have violence and in Chicago we have 40,000 abandoned buildings, unemployment among African American men is 50 percent right now it's a ridiculous situation and it's a moral situation. We need to understand now that violence is an epidemic in America, it must be stopped and we can't just sweep it under the rug because these young men and young men like them have to stop burying their friends."

Ricki then brought out Scooby's mother, Shirley who has lost all four of her children to gun violence in Chicago.

All of her kids were killed?

A story as tragic as Shirley's briefly made me wonder if there is a God at all. But when I thought about kids being murdered in cold blood, whether on the streets of Chicago or at a grade school in Newtown, I feel like there has to be a heaven so these angels have somewhere to go.

There just has to be.

"I did the best I could," Shirley said, wiping tears. "I was a single mom and worked hard day in and day out to make sure they had a roof over their head. I did everything a mother's supposed to do."

You can do everything right and still lose it all.

McMillan then started chiming in on how we can prevent these tragedies from happening in the future.

"The one thing parents have to do and this may sound cliché is they have to dare to love their children," he said.

Love your children...

"No police chief and no mayor can parent for us, we have to parent. We have to love our kids... Shirley loved her son. If the boy who killed her son had parents who poured that kind of love on him we might not be here today."

I grabbed a tissue to dab my eyes as I clicked the remote control and stopped on the local news. A snowstorm was on the way and all the newscasts were talking with dread about the impending "Snowpocolypse".

I used to be one of those reporters who got stuck on the "it's cold outside, back to you in the studio" stories. I found it to be such an insult to the viewer's intelligence. Of *course* it's cold here in the winter and of *course* it's going to snow and of *course* people are going to dig out their parking spaces and hold their spots with lawn furniture. It's not newsworthy – it's just part of living in Chicago.

"We've had snowfall 22 of the last 34 days in Chicago," the weather-man said.

Great.

When the weather report was over, it was back to the gloomy headlines.

194

"The baby that was born prematurely after both of his parents were killed in a hit and run car crash has died."

Everything's wrong in the world, back to you...

"The crash happened Sunday in Brooklyn New York after a BMW slammed into the livery cab carrying the young 21-year-old couple. They died but doctors managed to save their unborn baby at first. But it later died from sustained brain damage. The driver and passenger of the BMW abandoned the car after that crash."

I have a theory that only assholes drive BMW's. This news story definitely wasn't helping their image.

Enough of you, local news.

I continued to channel surf and landed on Dr. Oz who was talking about something called "Monkfruit" – a round fruit found in south east Asia that has 150 times the sweetness of sugar.

"I had a medical team do extensive research on this, and here's what they found," he said. "They found that traditional Chinese medicine has been using monkfruit for not decades but centuries."

I was now convinced that every working mother needed to watch Dr. Oz. I made myself a note to set a "series recording" of the show on my DVR so I wouldn't miss any future episodes.

I changed the channel from Dr. Oz and found myself unable to turn away from the traffic accident that was "The Bill Cunningham Show." Two sisters were on stage trying to be convinced by an expert to let go of the family feud. As I tried to figure out why they gave a talk show to a guy who looks like an elderly version of my son's dentist, I became entranced with the yelling match between the expert and one of the sisters named Yvonne.

Expert: "At some point, someone has to stop, right here, and say, 'From here on out it will be this way.'"

Yvonne: "I wish we could say that."

Expert: "You can."

Cunningham: "Yvonne listen up!"

Yvonne: "Some stuff that been done, the damage can't be undone!"

Cunningham: "Yvonne!"

Expert: "That's where forgiveness comes in."

Yvonne: "I do forgive her but I won't forget."

Cunningham: "Move on! Life is too short!"

Life is too short...These shows thrive on the walking wounded.

I turned off the television and fell asleep on the couch. Yvonne from "The Bill Cunningham Show" was in front of me in my medicine-induced dream, looking bewildered.

"You've got to get the help you need," I said. "Otherwise, you will just continue the cycle. Don't you see?"

"I'm not doing no therapy!" Her yelling now escalated to a point of complete rage.

"Why do you think it's a bad thing? It can help you feel good about yourself."

She frowned, and tried to think of a retort. Suddenly she put her head in her hands and started to wail. I went over to her and hugged her as she had a deep cry.

As I rocked her I heard,

Everyone who is mean is one deep breath away from tears. We have to love them all...

And with that statement, I woke up.

We have to love them all.

⚜ ⚜ ⚜

CHAPTER THIRTEEN
JOHN OF GOD

Facebook Status: So I just got a text from phone number I don't recognize saying "test". And I wrote back "who is this?" and they said "God."?!

✣ ✣ ✣

In the weeks after my meeting with Gail Thackray, I'd started compiling research about healer John of God. Not only had he been featured on the major networks, but Oprah Winfrey was working on a special about her trip to visit him in Brazil for OWN.

One of the clips I found on Youtube was from a documentary that followed John of God from 2003-2005. Dr. Jeffrey Rediger, a psychiatrist and physician from Harvard Medical School, goes to Brazil to witness the surgeries John of God performs without using anesthesia or sterilization. From eyes being operated on with small knives, to tumors being removed from breasts and brains, Rediger was shocked by what he saw.

"I have to change the way I think about the world," he says, after watching a tumor being taken out of a man's shoulder.

As Rediger watches John of God cut into a woman's cornea with a small knife, and again, using no anesthetic and no sterilization, she doesn't even wince.

"I can't explain that," he says in the documentary. "I've heard some people use the term 'spiritual anesthesia.' I have no way to understand that."

There's a scene in the documentary where Dr. Rediger speaks of understanding this phenomenon in his head, but not accepting it in his heart. Shortly following that statement, a stain appeared on his shirt. He was suddenly bleeding from a small incision over his heart. The locals see this often, and call it an "invisible physical surgery". He bled for an hour.

Oprah then interviewed Rediger on her network show before it went off the air and he still had trouble putting his experience into words.

"This guy (John of God) has a second grade education, and I do have to say, these are things that I don't understand, and so I can't fully endorse things that are beyond my understanding but I've seen them happen," he told Oprah.

"I think the powers of belief, the power of the mind are far more powerful than we have even begun to explore, I think that's an unexplained wilderness in terms of research."

He then admitted that his visit to Brazil turned his life upside down because everything he thought to be true in his medical training was now being questioned by the practices of John of God.

"Do you consider yourself a religious person?" Oprah asked.

"Because of this, I am actually more interested in the development and cultivation of a spiritual life," he responded. "There is something that settled in my heart ... that I feel that I know something true."

"What is it that you know that is true?"

"What I really believe is that we really do matter, more than we have a clue about – every one of us does. There's something irrefutable and good about who we are. We often may feel alone but we're not alone in any way like we believe we are. We are more connected than we believe. There's a dignity and goodness to what we bring into the world. And the point of our life is to somehow begin to get it about that."

I sent the different links from Youtube to some friends and suggested a "girls trip" to Toronto. The only man in my life continued to be Britt, and I figured a weekend away was short enough to be do-able.

"Anyone up for seeing this woo-woo healer man?" I wrote.

Therese was already considering a trip to Brazil to see John of God, so Canada was a no-brainer. My friend Amber wanted to join too.

As the weekend was approaching, we received emails from Gail about how to prepare. Anyone attending had to wear all white. (This included underwear, bras, socks, shoes. Everything.) The "healing entities" request the white attire.

Entities?

We could bring photos with us of loved ones we wanted to be blessed or healed by him, and we were to write down our intentions or "prayer" and have it in our hand when we see John of God. Everyone would get a chance to be seen, but because there were hundreds if not a couple thousand people attending the event, the time would be brief.

"Maybe you'll meet a hot, spiritual guy there," my friend said. "This trip could change your life."

The night before my flight, I was packing in a fury; and as I tried to find white clothes, I realized I had nothing that would work for cold weather. The only white things I had were shorts, capri pants and short sleeve shirts.

Nobody in the Midwest wears white when it's snowing!

I threw the capris into my suitcase along with a light beige wrap and an off-white sweater. I was anticipating a breeze.

I hope the white entity police don't get upset.

The only white shoes I had were sandals, so I dug up some worn out running shoes that I believe were white at one time, and threw them in my bag along with some white running socks.

An old colleague once told me, "Always dress your best on an airplane. You never know who you will run into."

While I usually like to abide by this rule, on the Friday morning I was heading to Toronto, everything was going wrong. The weather was terrible, which means traffic is going to suck, and there was a deadly accident on the expressway blocking all lanes on the road I needed to take to get to the airport.

I skipped the shower, threw on some yoga pants and left.

So of course I get seated next to a really hot guy in business attire.

Shit!

Then, as I was checking into the hotel in Toronto, I heard a familiar voice.

"Just call me Erich," said the man to the woman behind the counter. I was staring at Erich "Mancow" Muller – a radio and TV "shock-jock" from Chicago.

I picked the wrong day to look like a bum.

"Fancy seeing you here," I said. I've known Mancow for years. While he acts tough and heartless on the air, deep down, he's a very spiritual guy. (I just wish he wasn't afraid to show this side on the radio.)

"Hey there, Jen!" He said in a slightly "Oh shit, I've just been busted by a fellow Chicagoan for being at a healing conference" kind of way.

Mancow is also friends with Gail who is a frequent contributor to his show.

"You know, I was just on the phone with William Shattner and I invited him to this thing," Mancow continued. "But he wasn't buying it."

I could just see Shattner showing up in all white joining John of God on the stage.

"Beam me up, Johnny!"

"I'm here because Gail just raves about John of God," I said. "I'm kind of curious."

Mancow played down his desire to meet John of God, even rolling his eyes at the thought of "being healed." But I found it hard to believe that he'd fly to Toronto if he thought it was all a bunch of crap.

As we chatted, several people walked by in their white attire.

"Did you pack your white clothes?" I asked.

"Oh yeah," he said. "But you know, I'm a Christian, and all this talk about 'entities' wanting you to be in white. Entities? That's freaky, right? What's that about? I mean come on, did you have to wear white to meet Buddha?"

He had a point.

We parted ways and I decided to wander the grounds. While this was a three-day event, people could buy passes to each individual day or get the three-day pass. I didn't feel like I could stand three days of anything, so I bought tickets to the Saturday and Sunday events. Amber did the same. Therese wanted the full experience, so she had arrived earlier that morning to be present for all three healing sessions. I called her room but she didn't answer.

Maybe she had a "surgery"?

The way Gail explained it, getting chosen for a psychic surgery is "the greatest honor." In Brazil, you can have either hands-on surgery (complete with the weird looking knife and no sterilization or anesthetic) or psychic surgery, where you sit in a chair and these so-called "entities" do their thing. By law, John of God isn't allowed to do the hands-on operations outside of Brazil. He can, however, do the "psychic" surgeries on the road.

There were people in wheelchairs and others using walkers for support. I didn't have any illness that I knew of so I wasn't there to relieve a physical ailment. I did, however, want some relief from the sadness in my heart.

I noticed a group wandering the halls lugging cases of water with John of God's face on it.

Apparently John of God had gone commercial.

Figures.

I got to the main hall and saw several hundred empty chairs set up in front of a stage, and various vendors selling crystals, dvd's, cd's, books and jewelry. The events of the day had finished and everything was closing up. It looked like a street fair that had been kidnapped by a concrete tower. Everything felt very corporate – not how I'd picture something for a man who claims to heal the ill.

"Excuse me, have you seen Gail?" I asked one volunteer.

"I believe she's at the check-in," he said.

I continued to search but came up empty. I went back to my room and found a message from Therese. She said she had "psychic surgery" and needed to sleep for the next several hours.

What does that mean?

When Amber arrived, we decided to have a quick bite to eat and then go to bed early. The line would be forming at 6 a.m. and we wanted to be well rested.

Have you ever had an experience where all you want to do is doze off, yet no matter how hard you try, you can't fall asleep? Amber and I tossed and turned all night. When the alarm went off, we both felt as though we'd gotten about 15 minutes of shut-eye.

"This sucks," Amber said.

"I need coffee," I groaned.

I looked up and saw Amber getting dressed. She was wearing white jeans and a really nice white top.

Even on no sleep and with no shower, she looked gorgeous. (If I didn't know how nice she was, I would hate her for this.)

I wiggled into my capris. Not only were they skin tight, but they were shorter than I'd remembered, falling just below the knee. My thighs felt like sausages being smashed into their casing.

Fabulous.

Worried that I'd be cold, I put on my pair of gym socks. They were really thick and ugly, but they covered the areas where my capris were lacking.

"There," I said, pulling them as high as they would go.

I glanced down at my worn out tennis shoes, socks pulled to capacity and hip-hugging capri's. I looked like the kid in grade-school who got beaten up for dressing like a spaz. I grabbed my off-white sweater to wrap around my waste.

"Might as well complete the disastrous ensemble," I said. "If I did meet a hot guy, this outfit would definitely scare him off."

We went downstairs to check-in, got our tickets and waited in line. A few minutes later, I looked behind me and was shocked to see a friend from Chicago.

"Sheree?"

"Jenniffer?"

"Out of all these people, you stand behind me in line," I said. "What are the chances?"

"That kind of stuff always happens to you, Jen," Amber said.

Sheree then went on to tell us that she, too, had "psychic surgery" the morning before. She said she could feel something working on her eye while she was resting afterwards. She explained that she'd always had trouble with her one eye since she was a young child and that all night she felt as though there was activity and light around that eye.

"I slept all day yesterday," she said. "I only woke up to eat dinner."

"And you really think something happened to you?" I asked. Sheree is a very well respected life coach. She taught a class at the Chicago Tribune. While I knew she was spiritual, I would not have thought we'd be having a conversation about "psychic surgery".

"Oh I could feel it, yes," she said. "Absolutely. Even when I was sitting in the great hall before John of God came in, it sort of felt like something was playing with my hair. It was wild."

They play with your hair?

We went upstairs and ran into Gail in the great hall.

"We finally found you!" I said.

Gail looked at me and I could tell she couldn't place my face.

"It's Jenniffer Weigel from Chicago," I said. "Author of 'I'm Spiritual, Dammit?'"

"Oh yes!" She said, giving my outfit the once over. "I didn't recognize you."

When I interviewed Gail in Chicago, I was well rested and wearing a suit, not struggling to keep my eyes open with tube socks pulled up to my knees. I could see why I didn't look familiar.

"How do you feel?" she asked.

"We were up all night," I said. "And not by choice! We couldn't sleep."

"The entities wanted to keep you up so you would rest today after the surgery," she said with a laugh.

Entities have a sense of humor?

"Why don't you head to the triangles," she said. "There isn't a line yet."

On either side of the stage there were two wooden triangles, which is like the cross for John of God followers. Just as they do in Brazil, people say their prayers for loved ones in front of the triangles, and there is a basket next to them to leave pictures or pieces of paper with specific requests.

They say the baskets are then taken back to Brazil and put in a room where they are prayed over. There isn't really a time limit for how long you pray at the triangle. It's sort of an honor system. Most people seemed to have two or three pictures they put into the basket and then they stepped aside so the next person could approach. I had two pieces with me.

When just one woman was in front of me, I got a bit excited. But when five minutes went by, followed by ten minutes, I got pissed.

She didn't just have a few pictures – she brought an entire photo album. And she took out each and every one of them, said a prayer, and then placed it in the basket. Each time I thought she was done, another picture came out of the booklet.

I wanted to be the "triangle cop" and urge her to "MOVE" just like they do in rush hour, but I knew that raising my voice would not be welcomed in such a holy zone.

Hurry the hell up!

When she finally moved, I approached the triangle. I looked at my two pictures and said a prayer before placing them in the basket. Then I put my hands on the triangle and leaned my head into the center. As much as I tried to focus on my loved ones, all I could think was:

I wonder if the people behind me can see my panty lines.

I walked away and went back to my seat. It was only 6:45 a.m. and we had no idea when to expect John of God.

TWO HOURS went by, and there was no healer-man in sight. As the hall filled up, we heard musicians sing peaceful songs, and several people got on stage to tell their story in broken English about their healings in Brazil.

While I admit to being spiritual, this group was full of the stereotypes that give the new-age movement a bad name. The more testimonials I heard, the more I started to get antsy.

Maybe I can sneak away and look on my phone to get the score from last night's Blackhawks game?

In my second book, "I'm Spiritual, Dammit!" I have a chapter called "Don't Get Lost in a Guru." I describe how I was so passionate about a healer named Master John Douglas from Australia that I would panic if I left the house without his healing C.D.'s. I see this with many in the spiritual self-help arena – people get so lost in a healer or a religion that they lose sight of the power they have within.

I looked around the hall – hundreds if not a thousand people, all wearing white and waiting to see their healer, were praying with purpose. Was John of God their last hope? Would this experience give them relief? What if they didn't get their prayers answered? Would they give up?

Scanning the crowd, I saw Mancow. He seemed to be praying just like everyone else.

I wonder if he'll talk about this on the radio?

I could see how this experience would be enchanting if you were walking through beautiful countryside with sacred waterfalls and mountains such as the Casa in Brazil. But this concrete jungle in a Toronto hotel felt sterile and disconnected. I was starting to think that coming to this event was a really bad decision.

"This room has been blessed by John of God," the woman on stage said. "Keep your prayers in your heart and remember why you are here. Be sure to use this time to meditate and focus on your intention."

I was worried that if I closed my eyes, I'd fall asleep, so I did my best to stay alert.

Finally, at 9:15 a.m., John of God entered the hall.

We waited three hours for you. This better be good.

"Ladies and gentleman, welcome John of God!" said the woman on stage, bursting out of her white robe with excitement. The crowd cheered as people in the aisle reached out to touch John of God as he passed.

John of God was the "Elvis" of the spiritual guru world.

"I can't hear you," she screamed from the stage like a cheerleader for a football game. "Welcome to Toronto, John of God!"

He made his way onto the stage, and through an interpreter he spoke of his gratitude to all who were in attendance. He said he had been doing these healings for 56 years, and that Oprah Winfrey had been to the Casa and was airing a special on him the following day.

Really dude? Most of the people here have already consumed the Kool Aid. You don't need the sales pitch.

Then as he asked us to stand; he made an announcement that anyone who wanted a healing or surgery would receive it.

Anyone?

There was a collective gasp in the crowd. Apparently, this is highly unusual. The normal protocol is for each person to go before John of God, and he decides at that time if you are to be given "surgery". Here he was saying, "come and get it!"

A swarm of people started to line up against the wall.

"Do you want to go?" Amber asked.

"I was kind of hoping he would make that decision *for* me," I said.

"I want to go," she said, heading toward the line.

I followed her and watched as hundreds of very civil people started pushing each other like third graders to get a better spot in line. The man standing next to me looked like a professional athlete, but I couldn't place his name.

"You don't have to wait in this line," a woman said as she led him behind a white curtain.

I'd finally spotted an attractive man, and he was being ushered away. Apparently, he was getting the VIP treatment, which really pissed me off – kind of like when celebrities get free stuff. If there's anyone who should pay full price, it's the people getting paid millions of dollars. At a healing conference, the only people who should get taken to the front of the line are those in wheelchairs or the terminally ill. Not some professional athlete with rock hard abs.

As the line slowly moved closer to the entrance, a woman walked up and down shouting out information.

"If you are in this line, you are committing to a psychic intervention with John of God," she said.

She made it sound so … *weird*.

"This means no sex – with yourself or with others – no booze, no strenuous exercise and no spicy foods for 40 days."

Huh????

Amber and I looked at each other.

"No sex?" She gasped.

I wasn't dating anybody, so no-sex wouldn't be as much of an issue as an occasional glass of wine.

"Did she say 'no sex with yourself, either?" I asked.

I could see Amber doing the math in her head. She lived with her boyfriend, so 40 days of not getting any was gonna be challenging.

Sex or enlightenment?

"I'm still going ahead with it," she said.

The anticipation slowly built with each and every step as we got closer and closer to the white curtain. I looked over at Amber and her eyes were welling up with tears.

"I don't know what is happening," she whispered. "I feel like I'm going to start wailing."

Just before we went behind the curtain, a man put his hand on my arm.

"Take your black purse off your shoulder," he said. "No dark colors above the waist."

If these healing "entities" were going to fly overhead and somehow perform actual miracles, I found it hard to believe that the black strap on my shoulder would be a deal breaker. But I removed it anyway.

We turned left and there were people on either side of the line with their eyes closed, holding out their hands as if they were praying. We entered an area with a couple hundred chairs where people were sitting. Some had their hands in the air and some were holding crystals. I later found out they called this the "current room" where other healers or mediums volunteered to sit to "hold the space" for those getting the healing.

Where is John of God?

As we passed this group of "space holders" I suddenly felt a wave of emotions come over me, followed by goose bumps from the top of my head all the way to the tips of my toes. And before I knew it, I had tears streaming down my face just like Amber. I looked over and a woman was holding out tissues, almost on cue. Apparently, this uncontrollable weeping happens a lot at these things.

It was in that moment that I saw John of God up ahead. He was sitting in a chair, arms extended on the armrests and it seemed his eyes were closed. There were a couple of people on either side of him, also praying. Some people stopped to put their pictures or prayers in the basket in front of him as they went by. I paused as I stood before him and looked closely at his face. His eyes were rolling back in his head. I then felt an incredible wave of heat. It was as if I walked into a sauna.

Freaky!

I'd read that he doesn't remember the "psychic surgeries" because he's channeling different healers. I looked at him, said my prayers and continued to walk as directed. Unless you are pulled from the line, this is the protocol. (In Brazil, seeing John of God is free and you get to stop and ask him questions through an interpreter. In this setting, we needed to buy a ticket and couldn't even say "hi" to the guy.)

Bummer.

Exiting the John of God room, we were led to another area with a couple hundred chairs. As we took a seat we were instructed to put our right hand over our heart and pray for whatever we'd like to be healed.

My prayer was pretty simple: "Help me love myself unconditionally and tell my stories fearlessly." I figured if I could do those two things, everything else would fall into place.

"Keep your eyes closed," the woman standing in front of the crowd ordered when I took a peek at my watch.

At this point I was starting to wonder if this whole thing was just a bunch of crap. I tried to focus on my prayer, but after a few minutes my curiosity got the best of me and I opened one eye to see my surroundings. Across the aisle from me was a girl in a wheelchair. She had a breathing tube and seemed to be paralyzed. I looked to my right and there was a woman who'd lost all of her hair. Asking to "love myself" or to "tell stories fearlessly" suddenly seemed irrelevant.

Your have "princess problems" compared to these people, Jen.

As soon as every seat was filled, John of God came in front of the room. His eyes were still rolled back in his head as he mumbled something. I was now half praying and half looking for my iphone so I could record whatever words came out of his mouth. But before I could get the device out of my purse, he was finished. The interpreter mentioned something about how our prayers were healed in the name of Jesus; and then it was time to go.

The traffic cop came back to direct the group to the cafeteria where we were given a hand-out about our "post surgery protocol." Everyone gathered around tables in a haze as they read the rules aloud.

1. SLEEP UNTIL TOMORROW MORNING
2. NO EXERCISE OR STRENUOUS PHYSICAL ACTIVITY FOR 8 DAYS

3. NO SEX OR SEXUAL ENERGY (40 days if this is your first intervention.)
4. STITCHES REMOVAL. (A week from now you will be visited by the entities to remove your spiritual stitches.)

Spiritual stitches??

I had to read that fourth rule three times because I thought my eyes were playing tricks on me. We were then told we had to purchase 12 bottles of "blessed" water that would be our "prescription" for our specific surgery.

"In Brazil you would have been given an herbal prescription, but we couldn't bring those herbs here to Canada," the man said.

How am I going to get 12 bottles of water back to Chicago in my carry-on luggage?

My concerns over being scammed into buying "blessed" water were quickly interrupted by a sudden feeling of thirst, followed by hunger, and complete exhaustion. Before I could say "spiritual surgery" my head was bobbing like my Great Grandma Belva when she needed a nap.

"Wow, you are done, girl!" said my friend Sheree who was sitting next to me. "You're going to fall into your soup."

"Yeah Jen, you can't even keep your eyes open," Amber added.

What is happening to me?

"I think I need to go upstairs," I said, barely able to drag myself out of the chair.

Amber and I went back to the room and collapsed onto the beds. We slept for six straight hours. When we woke up, we had just enough energy to order room service.

"I don't feel like myself," I said, trying to sit up and comprehend how it was possible we slept until dinner.

After consuming our 30-dollar salads, we set the alarm for the next morning and went back to bed.

We slept through the night until the alarm went off at 5 a.m. Getting up, we were sluggish at best. I saw my capri's crumbled on the floor. I refused to put my thighs through the same kind of torture two days in a row, so I reached for the pair of beige pants I'd packed as a back-up and threw on my cream colored sweater.

"The entity police are going to have to come after me," I said, trying to keep my balance. I felt like I'd been sailing on a cruise ship for a week.

We went downstairs and ran into Gail at the elevators.

"How are you doing?" she asked.

"Dizzy and kind of sleepy," I said. "Is this normal?"

"Absolutely," she said. "I was out late with Mancow, so I'm pretty tired too."

"How is he liking all of this?" I asked.

"He had a psychic surgery. He was thrilled."

Say what?

"Then how did he go out last night? I couldn't keep my eyes open, let alone be social."

"He didn't drink and he'd slept all day," she said.

"What time do you think John of God will be coming in today?" I asked. "We waited three hours yesterday."

"You know, John of God is in the restaurant right now. You should go talk to him, Jen," she said.

"Now?" I gasped. My ultimate goal was to get an interview with John of God for my book, but there was no guarantee I'd be able to get him away from the conference. Now Gail was giving me permission to pursue a conversation and I was half awake and hardly "dressed to impress." These were not the circumstances I'd envisioned.

"Let's do it," Amber said, trying to give me confidence.

"He's just around the corner," Gail said.

I took a deep breath and headed into the restaurant as Amber followed. I scanned the room and saw a group dressed in white sitting in the corner.

There he is!

The remnants of eggs sat on a plate in front of him as he chatted and relaxed with his friends. Seeing him surrounded by his fellow healers, or "healing posse", I quickly got intimidated, but I approached him anyway.

"Hi John of God. My name is Jenniffer and I'm an author," I said reaching out my hand to greet him.

The interpreter let out an exhale that oozed "here comes another freaky fan" as he translated my words. John of God shook my hand, then Amber's. I tried to ask him a question – but nothing would come out of my mouth.

I've interviewed famous actors, politicians, you name it – and I've never been at a loss for words. There I was, standing in front of a farmer with a second grade education and I literally couldn't form a sentence.

"Uh, errrr, uh, fmmmb," I mumbled.

He looked at me with a blank stare.

"I'm a journalist from Chicago," I finally said. "You know, Oprah?"

Oprah?

"Ahhhhh! Oprah!" The whole table said.

Why did I bring up Oprah? Just being me isn't enough so I have to mention Oprah?!

"Oprah is airing a special on John of God," the translator said to me. "I believe it airs tonight."

John of God continued to talk, and the interpreter looked at me and said,

"He says to give Oprah a hug from him."

"Errr, OK." I groaned, knowing I had no plans to be seeing Oprah anytime soon.

Ask him about healing your heart, Jen!

I smiled, shook his hand again and tried to get up the nerve to talk. When I finally was able to create intelligible sounds, I said, "Thank you for being here. Thank you so much."

"Yes, thank you," Amber said.

We smiled, nodded, shook his hand, and slowly walked away from the table.

You asked him nothing!

The stroll back to the elevators felt like an eternity.

I turned to Amber and whispered under my breath, "I am so horrified. I want to crawl into a hole and die." Amber was staring straight ahead in a daze.

"Yeah, we weren't at our best," she said.

"Why did I freeze?" I put my head in my hands as we stood in front of the elevators. "Do you think he has some sort of psychic power where he shifts the electro magnetic field so people can't function? Because that was just weird."

"You should go back," Amber said. "Go back and ask the questions you wanted to ask. What's the worst thing that could happen?"

I could look like an even bigger asshole.

When I was a kid people would always approach the table where I'd be sitting with my dad and interrupt him to talk about sports because he was a sportscaster on television in Chicago. I hated those people for interrupting our time together. By going back to try and ask John of God my questions, I would become one of *those people.*

"I can't do it," I said, feeling terrified and unworthy.

My eyes filled with tears. All of my insecurities were bubbling to the surface and I had no way of stopping them.

"Sure you can," Amber said. "Let's just go back in there like we're looking for Gail and if he's still there, you can ask him your questions."

I tried to gather the courage to go back into the restaurant. After a few moments, I grabbed my iphone and hit "record" so I didn't have to worry about pulling it out if things went my way. We walked back toward the table and saw John of God talking to a young woman with the help of the interpreter. She'd pulled up a chair and made herself at home.

That's my seat!

"Forget it," I whispered to Amber. "Let's just go back to the conference hall."

My window of opportunity was now totally closed.

As we walked, Amber tried to talk me off the ledge.

"Look, what's done is done," she said. "Don't think about it. It's over. Maybe you'll get another chance to talk to him?"

I blew my one chance. I blew it.

We got in the line to re-enter the hall. There was a group of women standing in front of us swapping surgery stories.

"I met the sweetest man who said his chronic neck pain is totally gone," one of the women said. "I should have brought Michael here. His back has been a mess for years."

"Michael would NEVER come to one of these things," another woman said.

I looked around and saw couples holding hands as they waited in line.

I want to be with someone who would hold my hand in a place like this.

"There's a lady up in the front of the line showing pictures on her iphone of the scars her mother has from a psychic surgery on her hip," a woman said.

"Oh I know," her friend said. "And the daughter is a surgeon. She's totally blown away."

I'd heard all sorts of "hard to believe" stories since my arrival at this event, but nothing that seemed to offer proof. I decided to stop feeling envious of the loving couples in line and pulled out my iphone. The journalist in me was back in the game.

"Excuse me," I said, leaning in to the group. "Did you just say a woman had scars and there's a picture of this?"

"Yes," she said. "She's at the front of the line. Come here, I'll take you to her."

The woman took my arm and started leading me to the front of the line. I didn't even have time to compute how odd it was that a person I didn't know was now taking me to another person I didn't know with possible proof of "magical scarring".

"Here," my tour guide said, putting me next to a beautiful woman who was proudly sharing photos with the crowd from her phone.

"She just woke up suddenly at about three this morning and said she felt something happening in her hip, so I turned on the light, and when I saw this, I said, 'Mom, I have to take a picture! I can't even believe this.'"

I looked at the photo she was holding up and saw a very obvious scar that was at least three inches long.

"Did I hear that you are a surgeon?" I asked her.

"Yes," she said. This woman had a very serious look on her face. I got the feeling she was not a member of the "woo-woo" club by any means. "This scar looks like an incision that is about three days after stitches have been removed."

"And you're sure it wasn't there before she went to sleep?" I said, slightly overstepping my bounds.

"Oh I'm sure," the woman said.

She continued to stare at the image, as did everyone else within 10 feet of her phone.

"Have you had anything odd happen to you since you've been here?" I asked her.

"Not really," she said. "I mean I've been tired, but I haven't seen anything too out of the ordinary. Not until I saw this."

I walked back to my spot in line.

"What did you see?" Amber asked.

"A scar. She said her mom felt something working on her hip in her sleep."

"I felt something working on me too when I was sleeping," she said.

"You did?"

I had no scars and had experienced nothing out of the ordinary other than my extreme sleepiness.

Are they making this up?

"Be sure you write down everything you want on your piece of paper when you go before John of God," one of the women in front of us said. She was obviously the seasoned veteran of the group, arming her friends with a list of her version of "best practices". "Then you hold that in your hand when you put your right hand over your heart."

"We're supposed to hold our prayers in our hand after we see John of God?" I quietly asked Amber. "I thought we were supposed to have it on hand when we walked before him, and that was it?"

I hate all these rules!

"And don't be afraid to ask for what you really want," the woman continued. "God loves you that much. He wants you to have all that you ask for and more."

I had wants just like everyone, but I was torn between praying for my highest good, or praying for stuff.

"Caroline Myss says, 'we have no idea what's for our highest good except God.' But then there's Gail's theory that we all deserve the ability to attract abundance with ease. Am I supposed to write, 'I want a bigger house for me and Britt' on my piece of paper, or is that not spiritual?"

I'm so confused.

"I'm praying for my highest good, because sometimes I might not know what's best for me," Amber said.

Hearing Amber, the woman in front of us turned around and said, "I'm cautious of that 'highest good' prayer though, because the 'highest good' could be a lot of work. I'm looking for ease in my life."

"Shit, she has a point," I said to Amber. I was exhausted. Did I really want to be a spiritual warrior? "I like the sound of 'easy.' Maybe I better rethink this."

⚜ ⚜ ⚜

We walked into the hall and got seats closer to the front.

Assuming that John of God wouldn't be arriving for a couple of hours, we did our stop at the triangle to pray for our loved ones and went back to our seats to meditate. I've always sucked at meditating. Rather than focusing on "nothingness," my mind wanders aimlessly and I start beating myself up for not being able to focus on the proper stuff, which according to most gurus is nothing.

I sat for what seemed like an eternity in my chair, praying and trying not to let my "to-do" list enter my brain.

Finally, at 9:20 a.m. John of God came down the aisle for his welcome. Once again, he waved to the crowd and made it to the stage. Seeing him was a painful reminder of how much I blew it during our meeting just two hours earlier.

You come all the way to Toronto and are given a gift of talking to this guy and you blow it. What is wrong with you, Jen? How could you do that?

While listening to my inner monologue it was obvious I still really needed to work on loving myself.

As he addressed the crowd, John of God didn't bother with the sales pitch, or talk of the Oprah documentary. He mentioned how high the energy was with the group and that more psychic surgeries would be available to anyone who felt a calling.

Anyone?

I looked over at Amber to see if she was game.

"Totally," she said.

"Does this mean we have to buy 12 more bottles of water and go without sex for 80 days instead of 40?" I mumbled as we headed toward the line.

Our placement in the hall got us a pretty good spot as we waited to enter the area where the healings took place. We dutifully took our dark purses off our shoulders and moved single file as directed.

A different group of people stood on either side of the line holding out their hands and praying as we walked by.

Is this really going to make a difference?

"Trust," one of the women said to me right on cue as I walked past.

Gotcha.

I felt much more relaxed about the whole thing the second time around. Knowing what to expect, I was able to take my "reporter" hat off, which allowed me to be more present. I still wasn't completely convinced this experience would really heal anybody, let alone me, but I kept moving.

As we filed past the "current room" I felt a surge of emotion come over me as it had the first time. Both Amber and I were crying, and before we could think, "I need a tissue," someone handed us a box of Kleenex.

We got into the room where John of God was sitting on his throne-like chair. Instead of looking like a demon possessed, this time, he had a soothing smile. He looked each and every one of us in the eye. While I liked this much better than the eye-roll thing, it did make me wonder, "is he channeling a nicer healer or is he just phoning it in today?"

Maybe he was out late with Mancow.

We took our seats in the next room and waited for John of God to come in. The woman at the front of the room told us to put our right hands over our hearts and think of the healing we'd like to have. I took my piece of paper with my prayer and put it in my hand, and then placed it over my heart.

Just surrender, Jen. Surrender to whatever comes next.

I took a deep breath, closed my eyes and felt extreme warmth over my entire body. The area over my left breast was also very hot, as if I'd stuffed a heating pad in my bra.

Is this in my mind?

Rather than try to find my phone to record John of God, I kept my eyes closed as directed and focused on my breathing.

I am open to this healing. I am open to this healing.

The warmth on my left side continued the entire time I was seated. The woman in front of the crowd continued to say prayers from the Bible. Since John of God is Catholic, (and I was raised Protestant – sort of) most of the prayers and references were very familiar. My mind was so focused on my heart that I didn't know if I'd been sitting there for five minutes or an entire hour when John of God finally entered. With his eyes still open, he stood in front of the room and announced that we all received our requested healings.

Are you sure?

We stood up and were led out to the cafeteria for the "post surgery" briefing. Since we'd already sat through the tutorial the day before, Amber and I went in the other direction.

"How do you feel?" I whispered.

"Pretty good. You?"

"Good!" I said. "I don't feel any of the exhaustion I felt yesterday. I feel energized."

We wandered over to the tables where they were selling crystals, and sort of lingered in the great hall where several hundred people were still sitting, hoping to be seen by John of God. A woman was on stage singing songs as we stood in the back and listened.

"I wonder where Therese is?" I said as I studied the crowd.

"Are you hungry?" Amber asked.

"Not really. You?"

"No."

We both stood there like two zombies.

"Maybe we should go back to the room," I said.

"Good idea." Amber was beginning to look tired.

"We come all the way to Toronto and we only see the inside of this hotel," I said. "We might as well be in Detroit."

By the time we got back to the room, that tired feeling we'd experienced the day before had returned.

"I'm putting on my bathrobe," I said, anxious to collapse.

I grabbed the hotel robe and went into the bathroom to change. As I looked in the mirror, I thought I saw faint markings on the left side of my chest.

Must just be wrinkles from my bra.

But as I looked closer, I realized, these weren't wrinkles. I rushed out of the bathroom to show Amber.

"Is it my imagination or do you see something here?" I asked, showing her my chest.

"Holy shit!" she screamed. "Those look like incisions!"

Incisions?!

Just above my heart were two visible lines, and one very faint line that looked like a stitch across the more prominent markings. We immediately took out my phone to take a picture.

"So these are really here, right?" I said to Amber, still not believing my own eyes.

"Oh they're here alright," she said. "I need to get a better camera though."

Amber reached into her bag and got out her professional camera.

"Get over here by the window so I can use natural light."

I stood there motionless as Amber clicked away, and thought back to the first documentary I saw on John of God with Dr. Jeffrey Rediger, the psychiatrist and physician from Harvard Medical School. After watching John of God perform healings, Dr. Rediger had a small mark over his heart that wouldn't stop bleeding and didn't know what to make of it.

While I wasn't bleeding, I was now looking at red lines that weren't on my skin prior to my walking in front of John of God that morning. They say physical markings will show up for those who need proof of a healing.

I remembered Dr. Rediger's words:

"I think the powers of belief, the power of the mind, are far more powerful than we have even begun to explore."

Did I make these markings show up because I wanted them to?

After the photo session, I felt so much heat coming from my heart it was making my chin hot.

"Does it feel hot around here?" I asked Amber, pointing to my chest.

Amber put her hand over the left side of my chest and pulled it back like she'd just touched a hot stove.

"Shit," she said. "Yes. That's very hot."

"So I'm not dreaming this?" At this point, I didn't know if I was experiencing something truly unique or just suffering from exhaustion.

"This is happening," she said.

I got into the bed and reclined. My left upper chest felt like a pot of boiling water was resting on my boob.

This is really fucking strange.

"Are you feeling anything weird?" I asked.

"No. Just sleepy again."

I looked over at the clock as I was dozing off. It was 10:15 a.m.

We didn't look at the time again until 2:30 that afternoon when we woke up to the sound of Therese knocking on the door.

"Hey," she said, coming in with her luggage. It would be time to head to the airport in a couple of hours and we all felt like we'd been woken up in the middle of the night.

"Let me see your markings," Therese said. Amber had left her a message that we saw something on my chest. I pulled back my robe all to find the lines had faded away.

"I've got the pictures," Amber said, going to get her camera.

"I have to tell you about how I blew it with my John of God meeting," I said, trying to sit up in bed.

"You MET John of God?" Therese gasped.

"Well, if you can call it that."

I then told her all about how I tried to talk to him, and that I walked away humiliated without asking a single question.

"I felt so stupid."

"That was divine," Therese said.

"Me feeling like an idiot was divine?"

"Yes," she said. "You asked to heal your heart, right?"

"Right."

"So you were intersecting with John of God so he could bring up all your insecurities and fears and pain and all of the suffering that's come from that in this lifetime and all the other lifetimes, so that when you went in for the healing everything was on the table and you were ready. Then they could heal your heart at the level you had asked for from the beginning. And it took you having that encounter with John of God to do it. This went pretty deep."

"So I was supposed to blow it?" I asked.

"Yes, because you are loved unconditionally. So clap your hands and say, 'thank you for the healing. Thank you John of God for coming to Toronto,'" Therese said as Amber showed her the pictures from her camera. "From the looks of these, it seems like you got your surgery. Now the healing can begin."

⚜ ⚜ ⚜

At the airport in Toronto, I opened my emails and found a link that a friend had sent me of Oprah's blog explaining her visit with John of God.

JENNIFFER WEIGEL

She wrote about standing in front of him as he cut open a woman, which almost made Oprah pass out.

"I thought, yes, *that is a real knife, and yes, that is real blood dripping down her white pants. How is that happening without anesthesia, without her even flinching?*"

She then went on to talk about the extreme heat she felt in John of God's presence:

"As I watched, my fingers got hot. Heat rose through my arms and chest until I felt like I might implode. *Is my body bursting? Am I passing out?* I told myself to think calm thoughts. But I felt like I might actually throw up – on camera. *I've got to get to my chair. If I can make it there, I can steady myself...*"

Somehow, reading Oprah's blog made me feel less crazy. While I didn't see John of God cut open a woman's chest, I'd still experienced something I couldn't quite put into words.

She felt the heat too. What was with that damn heat?

My brain was racing. How would I be able to interpret this whole trip to my friends and loved ones?

How?

Flying home was a bit more complicated than the trip there because I now had to lug a case of water in a second piece of luggage. I had some explaining to do when I was going through customs.

The agent picked up one of the bottles and looked at the image of John of God.

232

"So what brought you to Toronto?" he asked, turning the bottle as he read the label.

"I went to a healing conference," I said.

"And what are these?" he asked, taking a good look at John of God's picture.

"That is blessed water from a guy named John of God," I said, slightly embarrassed. "Have you heard of him?"

The man looked at me with a slight smile. "No, I haven't."

He lifted a couple more bottles, looked at them closely, and put them down. At first I was worried he would be condescending, but after a couple minutes he seemed to be genuinely concerned.

"So you think that if you drink this water, it will heal you?"

"Well, um, I'm not sure because I've only had a few sips," I joked.

He had a sweet face with large dark brown eyes. He took a long, hard look at my passport.

"You know what I think?" he asked.

"What do you think?" I asked, smiling.

"I think you could buy water at home, and bless that water, and say, 'Heal me, water,' and that will work just the same."

That would have been a lot more convenient.

"Because at the end of the day, the only healer I think we need is ..." and he pointed to the sky. "The one up there. That's it."

He looked me in the eye.

"I had a brother who was told by a doctor that he only had a few months to live," he started to explain. "But you know what? He went on to have three kids. So they don't know! Doctors don't know everything. Only he knows," he said, pointing up.

"Everything seems to go back to that guy, doesn't it?" I said.

"Only *he* knows. You have a great rest of your day," he said putting down my bottles.

"Thanks. You too."

I gathered my water, put it in my second bag, and slowly rolled it out of the terminal.

⚜ ⚜ ⚜

CHAPTER FOURTEEN
TEARS IN MY TIRAMISU

Facebook Status: "Let the tears come. Let them water your soul."
-Eileen Mayhew

❧ ❧ ❧

Re-entry into the real world after my John of God weekend was odd. I felt like I had incredible clarity, yet I couldn't find the words to explain to anyone what had happened to me.

Amber was having a similar experience.

"I went clubbing with some friends, and I felt like I was out with a bunch of monkeys," she told me over the phone a few days after our return. "People think I'm so weird for not drinking. They just don't get it."

"How's the no-sex thing going?" I asked.

"That isn't as hard to explain as the water bottles with John of God's face on it," she laughed. "How about you?"

"I was watching Showtime and had to turn it off because the movie was getting too racy," I said. "I didn't want to get all riled up and then not be able to do anything about it."

"I have a bachelorette party to go to this weekend," she said. "I don't know how I'm going to do this!"

"You'll find a way," I said. "We didn't lug all that bottled water back here to not succeed!"

"You going to be around tonight?" she asked.

"I'm going to get dinner with Billy," I said. "I'll call you after I get home."

While most people know Billy Corgan for being the frontman of the band the Smashing Pumpkin's, he's also a poet, a wrestling fanatic and the owner of a tea shop called Madame Zuzu's in the Chicago suburb of Highland Park.

The first time we had tea, I walked in to meet him at Zuzu's and the music stopped me cold in my tracks.

Virginia?

The familiar sounds of Vaughn Monroe and his orchestra were playing through the sound system.

My grandmother Virginia and her sisters sang and traveled with Vaughn Monroe in the 30's and early 40's. While Vaughn was quite a crooner in his era, he's not exactly a household name these days. I put my coat and purse down at a table and approached the young man behind the counter.

"Do you know if this is satellite radio?" I asked.

"No this is Billy's personal ipod," he said.

"I swear this is my grandmother singing right now," I said. "Can you please look at the ipod and tell me if this is Vaughn Monroe?"

The guy walked over to the music system and read what was displayed on the screen.

"It says Vaughn Monroe and his orchestra, yep," he said.

Holy shit!

When Billy walked in a few minutes later, I practically tackled him.

"You like Vaughn Monroe?!"

"I'm obsessed with Vaughn Monroe," he said.

"My grandmother sang with him and his orchestra with her sisters," I said. "I swear she was singing when I walked in."

"Well I have about 1500 songs on that ipod," he said.

"And I just happen to walk in during the three minutes where a Vaughn Monroe song is playing with my Granny singing?"

That's weird.

A few minutes into our conversation, another Vaughn Monroe song started to play.

"You've got to be kidding me!" I said. "Do you have a remote control under the table or something that's making this happen?" I asked, looking around for a secret device.

I soon discovered that Billy and I had more in common than Vaughn Monroe. He's incredibly intuitive, and was in the process of writing a spiritual memoir.

"I've been writing it for four years," he said.

Billy admitted he was suffering from writer's block, so when I visited John of God, I added his name in the basket of prayers to see if it would help him finish the book. When I put his name in the basket, I looked at my watch and made a mental note of the time. It was 7:23 a.m. in Toronto. Billy was on tour in Texas, which is one hour behind.

We met for dinner after my return so I could tell him about my experience. I was pretty amazed to hear his version of what happened that day:

"I woke up and it was 6:23 and I felt like a distinct presence come over me and I asked myself 'What is that?' and realized, 'Oh I bet it's the John of God healing' and my ears started really ringing. Then I just put myself in a meditative prayerful state and tried to receive what was coming, I asked, 'Who's working on me?' and a voice said 'St. Francis of Assissi.' I didn't know that was one of John of God's angelic guides and I asked what was happening and the voice said they are 'deactivating the virus. ' And I understood it as a helix reorganization was going on. I just put myself in a meditative state and tried to receive it. It lasted maybe five minutes."

"That's really incredible," I said, realizing this was probably the first time I'd heard someone use "helix reorganization" in a sentence.

"How are you feeling since being back?" he asked.

"It's kind of hard," I said. "It's very lonely at times because I still feel like I had this incredible experience that is so hard to explain. And I'm noticing that some of my friendships and relationships are shifting. A few people think this is really cool, and others think I'm totally nuts because I won't even have a sip of wine."

"That makes sense because of the work you've been doing on yourself," he said.

He then explained how my shift in energy could be compared to a chord in music. He talked about music vibrations and their capacity to heal. If you have a chord that is harmonious, where each note creates a certain vibration, and a note in that chord goes up, the other notes need to shift to stay in harmony.

"Your note, or vibration went up. So their notes either need to go up or go down. They can't stay the same. If they do, the chord will no longer be in harmony."

❧   ❧   ❧

A couple of days later, I was assigned to emcee a Tribune class called "Life After Divorce" with syndicated columnist Amy Dickinson and dating coach Bela Gandhi.

Before the event got started, I stepped into the bathroom. I heard two women walk in behind me as soon as I entered a stall.

"So are you ready to be enlightened?" One woman said this in a totally sarcastic tone.

"Yeah, right," her friend laughed. "Unless this class can teach me how to make a total prick who's skipped out on child support pony up instead of taking his new girlfriend to Miami, I don't think I care."

Oh shit!

I quickly exited the stall and washed my hands with lightning speed, keeping my head down in the hope that these women wouldn't recognize my face from the event poster in the hall.

I made my way back to the room and noticed several people coming in with a look of angst and panic.

I remember those days.

As things got started, I tried to put the group at ease by telling them a personal story.

"I want you to know that whether you're just starting down this divorce road, or if you've been on it for a while, things will get better," I said. "I personally tried to get back into the dating world too quickly. I thought it would help diminish the loneliness. What I discovered was that I was attracting people just like me who were also not quite healed. If you are wounded and you put yourself out there too soon, you will draw in someone with the same issues, and the two of you will be limping together trying to heal each others' wounds. This is being co-dependent and not in-partnership. You have to be whole – apart – before you can be whole with someone else."

Amy then shared that she was single for 17 years after her first marriage ended before she got remarried.

"When Bruno and I started dating, he said to me, 'What do you say we do everything differently?'"

Do everything differently...

"What do you mean by that, Amy?" A man near the back of the room asked.

Amy then explained that she and her husband went into their relationship with the intention to not make the same mistakes they had made in the past. From waiting to have sex, to putting their relationship before the needs of others, they were really choosing to lose the old patterns and "do things differently."

"Bruno will send me flowers every time I travel, which is so lovely; and this last trip I took, the bouquet was so gorgeous that I couldn't leave it in the hotel. I had to take it with me," she said. "So I wrapped the flowers up and I carried them on the plane, and you should have seen me with this big thing of flowers going through security! But the look on his face when he saw me coming toward him was just priceless."

"Thank you, Amy," the man who asked the question said, nodding his head and smiling.

If I could tell every man one trick that never gets old: Send flowers often and for no reason. It works wonders.

I looked out at the room and saw so many sad faces. The days of sending or receiving flowers for these folks were a thing of the past.

"Maybe you didn't want this divorce or you were cheated on," I said. "Whatever the reason for the divorce, it's OK to be angry and disappointed."

I thought of my friend John St. Augustine's words about forgiveness and shared them with the group.

"When you forgive someone, you're not condoning their bad behavior. You're setting yourself free. You're no longer a prisoner to your anger and resentment. It's a choice to stay mad. You can't change what happened but you can choose how you move forward. The healing can begin when you let go."

I noticed a woman sitting near the back shaking her head "no" as I spoke these words. At the end of the event, she approached me at the snack table. I had a feeling I was about to get an earful.

"Can I ask you something?" She said.

"Of course," I said.

"I submitted a question that you neglected to ask the experts," she said. The look on her face quickly turned from polite to "you've ruined my life."

"I asked all the questions on my list," I said.

"No you didn't," she said, raising her voice. "I sent my question in ahead of time."

This woman's question involved an ex-husband who was gay, but he was now dating other women. She wanted to know if it was her duty to let those women know that he was gay. She also wanted to tell her children about their dad's sexuality.

"We combined your question with another very similar question," I explained.

"That's not helpful!" She screamed. The woman was now so close to my face that I was able to see she was wearing violet colored eyeliner.

It really brings out her eyes.

I looked over my shoulder and realized both Amy and Bela were still in the room, talking to other attendees.

"I am happy to bring Bela and Amy over here," I said.

"No, they're busy," she said, shaking her head. "They don't have time to answer my question."

"They're not too busy to walk over here if you just ..."

"NO!" She interrupted.

I took a deep breath and put my hands on her shoulders.

"I am telling you that I can offer you a solution and get your question answered, and you don't want to hear it," I said. "Do you want to have your question addressed or do you just want to yell at someone?"

Sometimes people really don't want to have their problems solved. They merely want a platform where they can bitch. And I was not willing to stand there and be this woman's punching bag.

She stood there silently as I brought Amy and Bela over to meet her. As I turned around, a different woman was waiting to ask me a question.

"Jenniffer, my son's wife left him for a man she thought was a billionaire and now she's found out he's actually a con artist and totally broke; so now she will only let me see my grandchildren if I pay her money," she said.

Whaaaaaat???

"How can I have a relationship with my grandchildren without being blackmailed?"

I think there's a special place in hell for people who use their children as negotiating tools when they're getting divorced.

"Where is your son?" I asked, thinking I could get the full story from him directly.

"He's not here," she said. "I told him I would come so I could take notes."

As parents we like to try to fix our children's problems by doing the work *for* them.

"Is he getting any counseling for this?" I asked.

"SHE left HIM," she insisted.

"I understand that, but even if we're not the one who wants to get divorced, therapy is still a good idea," I said.

"He works about 60 hours a week," she said. "He's a physician."

SO?

"I still recommend it," I said.

I noticed Amy walk away from the crabby lady. Whatever advice Amy had given her, it was obvious it wasn't what the woman wanted to hear. Bela tried to calm her down and took her aside. Eventually, the woman left in tears.

"How long ago did her husband leave her?" I asked Bela as we got in the elevator.

"Eleven years ago," she said.

ELEVEN YEARS?!

As my mind started to slip into judgment mode, I thought of my own grudge against my father's father, Grandpa John. He'd been dead for over a decade before I could even consider letting go of my anger over his behavior. I was really no different than this woman, who was probably in a puddle of her own tears in some parking garage in downtown Chicago.

"I hope she can let it go," I said.

Let it go.

⚜   ⚜   ⚜

The next morning I was heading to a restaurant to have break-fast with two women from my neighborhood. They said they wanted to hear all about my John of God experience, but as soon as I sat at the table, it was obvious they had another agenda.

"So what's the deal, Jen? Are you dating anyone?" Dana asked.

"No," I said.

My friends had done everything in their power to try and set me up, or get me back on Match.com, and I had been resisting for months. Now, they'd come to their own conclusions.

"Either there is a secret guy in your life you aren't telling us about, or you're gay," Mary said.

"I'm not gay," I said.

"Then who's the secret guy?" Dana said, half kidding.

I sat there in silence.

"I KNEW it!" Mary said.

"Why haven't we met him?" Dana asked.

"Because he doesn't live here," I said.

"So how often do you see each other?" Dana asked.

"Maybe every couple of months," I said.

"That's not a relationship," Mary said.

"I sort of like it this way. I'm so busy with work and Britt that I couldn't really handle someone here full time."

"That's what you're telling yourself," Mary continued. "But the reality is, by being with this person, you are telling the universe that you only deserve a fraction of a man. Do you really want a fraction of a relationship?"

She made it sound so ... fractured.

"So do you mean to tell me that if a wonderful guy came around who was smart, employed, and crazy about you that you would say, 'sorry, I can only see you for dinner every couple of months'?" I don't buy it," Dana said.

"I really think I'm too busy for more," I insisted. "I feel more in control this way."

"Is your ex seeing anyone?" Mary asked.

"I don't know," I said.

"Usually you can tell by the way they dress," Mary said. "I knew my ex was getting laid when he started dressing like Justin Timberlake."

"Is the secret guy married?" Dana asked.

"He's separated," I said.

"That means he wants to have his cake and eat it too," Mary said. "He is controlling this relationship, not you."

"No he isn't," I said.

Is he?

Mary was a therapist, so her advice always held more weight than most of my friends.

"He tells you when he comes to town and you clear your schedule to see him," Mary said. "Plus he's still married. Doesn't sound like a lot of 'give-and-take' is happening here."

I knew she was right. I just didn't like to hear it.

I remembered Amy's words from our Life After Divorce event.

"When Bruno and I started dating, he said to me, 'what do you say we do everything differently?'"

"If you really want to find love, you have to stop settling for pieces of a whole," she continued. "The right person won't show up until you end this. It's like this dangling thread on your skirt that needs to be snipped off with the scissors."

Ouch!

"Don't give energy to the pieces that no longer serve you," Mary said. "You deserve better."

I deserve better ...

As I drove to work, a van cut me off in traffic. Before I could honk, I noticed it had a logo on the back window that read ANGEL.

I sped up to try to read what kind of business would be called ANGEL.

He's driving like an asshole, not an angel.

I tried to catch the van, but he was going 70 mph in a 45 mile-per-hour zone. He cut off a couple more people before I finally got behind him and could make out the words "ANGEL House Cleaning".

I was almost killed by an angel trying to clean house.

At that moment, my phone vibrated.

Is it you?

I'd been feeling some distance from my East Coast crush ever since my return from John of God. He didn't understand my "woo-woo" side, although he did a decent job of faking it.

I looked down and saw that it was my friend John St. Augustine checking in. I called him and decided to ask him for advice.

"I could really use a male perspective," I said.

I told him about my concern over not hearing back from my "secret guy".

"I think my visit to the healer man might have turned him off," I said.

"So this is interesting," John said. "You think he's backing off a bit, but do you really want to be with someone who doesn't embrace every side of you?"

"Well, no," I said.

"You are the most dynamic woman I know, and yet you are feeling insecure because you haven't gotten a text in a while? Forget it! You don't need to be going after anything, Jen. Just let it be."

"That's so much easier said than done," I said.

"I've seen you evolve and grow with this divorce and you're really digging under the hood, which is good. You're getting to the core of all these issues. We can mow the lawn and cut the weeds, but unless you dig into the dirt and get at the root, they will keep growing back. These insecurities are feeding the 'Old Jen.' The 'New Jen' needs to just trust, and the right person will come."

The right person will come ...

"You went to see John of God to bring forth Jen of God."

Jen of God.

"This is probably the most important time of your life. Don't feed the Old Jen with old behaviors. Otherwise, the same patterns will just show up. You are moving from who you used to be to who you are *going* to be."

"So by not feeding the old behaviors, that part of me will die because I'm not giving it fuel," I said.

"Exactly," he said. "This is what I call 'the curse of consciousness.' Not everybody takes this path and chooses to grow. But you have."

"Only 'New Jen' gets to eat at my table."

"Good. So when you do get the text from him, which will happen because you've had this awareness – and that's when things show up – think about this: when you do hear from him, you have to really make a choice. Are you going to go back to the old patterns, or are you going to choose differently?"

The following day, I had to give a book talk to a room full of women in their mid-80's.

After a buffet that included mushy pasta and garlic chicken, I stood in a corner and told a room of 40 very sweet great-grandmothers a variety of stories. From Dr. Mary Neal to Anita Moorjani, I felt that I had their complete attention. Due to the poor acoustics in the room, I had to shout for almost 45 minutes. When it was over I was exhausted.

As I got up to leave, the group's organizer handed me a bag.

"You have to take some Tiramisu with you," she said.

"Oh wow, you can't mess up Tiramisu," I joked.

"Sure you can," she said bluntly. "But they do a good job here."

I drove back to work with my high calorie dessert riding shotgun, and made a phone call that was long overdue.

Choose differently.

"Hey you," my East Coast crush said as he answered the phone.

"Hey you," I said, feeling nervous. "So, I've been thinking about a lot about things ..."

I then went on to tell him the story of how my friends accused me of either being gay or having a secret man. I told him that as much as I enjoyed spending time together, we probably shouldn't continue to see each other.

I sat in the silence wondering how he would respond. Part of me hoped he'd fight for me.

"No Jen, I can't be without you. I will come more often. I want you and nobody else!"

But that didn't happen.

"I understand where you're coming from," he said.

And while I know this was the mature response, it still sucked.

"Take care, you," I said, holding back tears.

"You too," he said.

I drove for several miles in silence. Even though I knew I'd made the right choice, it felt strange to "choose differently."

I wanted to go sit somewhere and look at the lake, so I drove several miles out of my way to a favorite spot.

Lighthouse Beach is a land of many "firsts". From my first Fourth of July fireworks display, to that first beer, there is not a segment of grass or grain of sand on that beach that hasn't been touched by my toes.

I parked my car and looked at the paper bag on my passenger's seat. I opened it up and found a fork, napkin, and tiramisu just begging to be eaten. I took the bag and walked out of my car to a bench that perches over the water.

My ex kissed my forehead right here. On our wedding day.

I zipped my coat to keep out the chill and pulled out my dessert. This was my place to be happy and alive. And now I was here feeling sad and alone.

As the memories of all the laughs and kisses and carefree moments came flooding into my mind, tears started streaming down my face. Eating cake while you're balling your eyes out is not easy. (It's hard to swallow food when you're chest is heaving with grief.) I cried so hard that a few drops fell into the foil container that held my treat. I looked at the moisture that was now trickling onto my food.

Your tears are falling into your tiramisu, Jen.

I set my dessert down and pointed my hands towards the sky.

"I give up, God. I give this whole thing up to you. Take this pain off my hands and help me."

I took my last bite and sat on the cold bench until I could no longer handle the chill. I felt full and empty at the same time.

✤ ✤ ✤

CHAPTER FIFTEEN
I LOVE YOU.
I'M SORRY.
FORGIVE ME.
THANK YOU.

Facebook Status:

"Do you have the patience to wait until your mud settles and the water is clear? Can you remain unmoving until the right action arises by itself?" Lao Tzu...

⚜ ⚜ ⚜

On day 32 of my "post John of God" 40 days, things were really starting to drag.

"How much longer do you have left?" My friend Jan asked.

"Eight days," I said.

"You got any big plans?" she asked.

"Well I kind of thought my life partner would've shown up by now. I don't know, day 20 would've been nice. So we could get to know each other for a few weeks, and then seal the deal on day 41 with a passionate romp."

"How'd that work out?" she asked.

"Not so great."

"How do you feel otherwise?" she asked.

"I seem to have a heightened sense of awareness, which is really cool."

"Yeah, you haven't had any alcohol in your system," she joked. "You have more brain cells than most."

I'd noticed my "Spidey senses" start to kick in at around day 15. If a problem came up, rather than call someone to help me talk through the issue, I simply got quiet, took a few deep breathes and the answer would come to me. It's as if someone took Windex to all of my interior windows and I was able to see clearly for the first time. My alignment seemed to be, um, really aligned.

"That's great," she said. "Any downsides other than no sex or booze?"

"Actually, yeah," I said. "I'm noticing that certain people who've hurt me in my past keep popping into my mind at the most random times. I'll be minding my own business, and the face of my first boss or the friend who disappeared when I got divorced just appear like a flash on a video screen. Some have actually shown up in my dreams."

"Weird," she said.

That night I went to dinner with Billy to catch up and get my mind off these haunting images. He picked a sushi restaurant appropriately named "Happy."

As we ordered, I started to share a story about my first stepmother Carol.

"My Dad was really into salt water fish and he had this huge 200 gallon tank," I explained sipping my miso soup. "Every weekend we would pick out new things to put into the tank. My step-mom was really jealous of how much time he spent with the fish. So one Sunday morning we woke up and everything in the tank was belly up. They were all dead. My Dad was devastated. He took the water to be tested and they found bleach. We think she poured bleach in the tank to kill the fish."

Billy looked in my eyes as he sipped his tea. His gaze was so intense it almost made me blush.

"How long ago was this?" He asked.

"About 1980," I said.

He looked at his wrist as if he was checking his watch.

"You gonna let it go anytime soon?" he asked.

"I'm not holding on to any anger," I said.

"Sure you are."

Am I?

"So, when does your fast end?" He asked.

Fast? What fast?

"Next weekend," I said.

"Oh, wow!" He smiled. "What are you going to do?"

"Well, I've been praying about it actually," I said.

Billy laughed as he put his hands together and looked up.

"Dear God, who should I have sex with?"

"Not quite," I said. "It's more like, 'Show me the next steps for my highest good and the highest good of all involved.' Whether it's with someone, or without, because I don't need a partner to be whole."

"Why do women have such a hard time admitting they want to be in a partnership?" He asked.

"Well, I have a theory that we need to love ourselves first before we can bring in the right partner," I said.

"Yes but that's putting the cart before the horse because I'm sure you've had 'bad' partnerships that were vital to you now even understanding what a 'good' partnership would be," he said.

"Sure. They helped mold me into who I am."

"We tend to classify partnerships as 'good' or 'bad' but technically speaking, if we're single, it means every partnership has been 'bad' because they've all failed," he said. "To me it's an evolving consciousness. Sometimes when I talk like this people think I'm being regressive. But for whatever reason we had a period where women had a particular place and men had a particular place and I think looking back now, those symbols – the guy with the Kools rolled up under his sleeve looking tough and Mrs. Cleaver in the kitchen – they seem a bit anachronistic. And I remember being part of the generation that destroyed those images because they were probably my parents. But we haven't replaced them with anything. All we've done is we've spent 40 or 50 years destroying those images and haven't really replaced them with a better version. We need to come up with integrated version. We've spent a lot of energy making fun of and humiliating the dad from 'Married with Children', or even Archie Bunker in his chair with the beer. The modern era has not replaced those symbols with something of equal or greater value. So in terms of spiritual integration, we want to take what we liked about Archie Bunker and what we liked about the tough guy and what we liked about Mrs. Cleaver and reintegrate it with what we've learned in the journey through feminism."

As Billy spoke, I tried hard to think of anything redeeming about Archie Bunker or Mrs. Cleaver.

"I've known way too many women in their late 30's and early 40's who are freaking out because they don't have babies," he continued. "Because they bought the missive that their career should come first. And they feel this gaping hole in their life because they didn't fulfill some part of their biological function which I would argue is part of your function – not to have children necessarily but to address the function that *tells* you to have children. I know people who decided *not* to have children and they're completely content and happy and I've known people who thought they didn't want to have children and they're lamenting what they lost in the exchange and they've turned their pet into their number one child. So there's something beautiful about the urge, something beautiful about a man's urge to dominate and there's something ugly about a man's urge to dominate. And there's something beautiful in a woman's urge to submit and something ugly about it too."

"I feel like after this healing, that I've gotten a scholarship to Harvard and I don't want to blow it," I said. "I really want to do things differently."

"I know a woman in Sedona who does soul re-patterning," he said.

There's a sentence you don't hear every day.

"Her name is Anne."

"A friend of mine connected me to someone who does that kind of work a few months ago," I said. "It wouldn't be Anne Emerson would it?"

"Yes, Anne Emerson," he said. "You know Anne?"

"Yes!" I said. "I was thinking I wanted to call her since I've gotten back. I can't believe you know Anne."

"Well, there's our 'connection' for this time," he joked.

That's weird!

Driving home, I thought about Billy's words.

"All we've done is we've spent 40 or 50 years destroying those images and haven't really replaced them with a better version."

Perhaps today's ideal woman could be some sort of hybrid between Phil Dunphy from the show "Modern Family" and the COO of Facebook, Sheryl Sandberg?

When I got to my house, I lit a candle in the living room and decided to try to meditate. I got centered in my comfy chair and took several deep breaths. As soon as I felt relaxed, my first stepmom popped into my mind, front and center.

AHHHHHH!!!

I tried to get neutral and took several more deep breaths. Then I brought in the big guns.

Hey God, help me understand why I'm seeing these images. Help me clear this from my mind.

Within minutes, a message started coming through loud and clear.

You asked to be healed, and you can't heal your heart until you forgive all the parts you've been avoiding. So let go of any resentments. Try to get to a neutral place with all those who have disappointed you or hurt you. No matter how big or how small. You have to let it go. This isn't condoning what they did. This is setting you free of the anger and the fear so you can be fully healed. Once you let go of this anger, you can fill your heart with love and trust.

The words were so super clear I wrote them down right away. One sentence kept replaying in my mind.

This isn't condoning what they did...it's setting you free.

Rather than letting go of the past, I'd apparently been pushing down my resentment into a deep dark tunnel of my subconscious.

Fill your heart with love and trust.

I looked on my coffee table and saw the title of the book Zero Limits, which was recommended to me by my friend Lisa Dietlin.

"This guy in Hawaii used a Ho'oponopono to help heal criminals," she said.

"Ho'oponowhato?" I asked.

"It's a kind of healing method in Hawaii that works miracles," she said.

In the book, author Joe Vitale traveled with a man named Dr. Ihaleakala Hew Len, who claims to be a master teacher of modern Ho'oponopono. Part of this Hawaiin technique includes saying, "I love you, I'm sorry, please forgive me, thank you," to clear away negative energy and heal any relationship or toxic situation.

The book claims that Dr. Len used this technique to help heal criminals in the Hawaii State Hospital by looking at their names in a file. He never even met his subjects. He just read their names while sending them love, forgiveness and gratitude.

I love you, I'm sorry, please forgive me, thank you.

"At first I kind of rolled my eyes when my friend told me about the book, "Lisa explained. "But I found myself on a Saturday morning so engrossed that I read it in one sitting. Now, I can simply think 'I love you, I'm sorry, please forgive me, thank you,' and it changes things. Former clients have returned, old friends re-entered my life and even negative beliefs have gone away simply by thinking and saying that mantra."

I got a pad of paper and wrote down every person I could think of who made my stomach turn.

Does the guy who cut me off in traffic last week count?

The act of creating this list was a great lesson in self-reflection. I had to be completely honest with myself. People I hadn't thought of in years found their way on to this piece of paper.

I took my list, looked at every name and said the words, "I love you, I'm sorry, please forgive me, thank you."

After I was finished, I felt a sense of relief followed by a feeling of accomplishment. I then decided that I would do this every day – either in the morning or at night, until I no longer felt that feeling of angst in the pit of my stomach.

I love you, I'm sorry, please forgive me, thank you.

⚜ ⚜ ⚜

The next night, I got a panicked call from a friend who had just gotten into a fight with her ex-husband.

"He's trying to move the kids to the suburbs and he's poisoning their minds against me," she said. "I also think he's going to get re-married and I hate this woman with a passion. I can't imagine her parenting my kids. I think I'm going to throw up."

I told her that she needed to try to do what I was doing.

"I know it sounds insane but just think of him and the new wife and say, 'I love you, I'm sorry, please forgive me, thank you,' I said. "See if it helps."

"You've gotta be kidding me," she said. "I don't think I'm capable of thinking of him and uttering those words at the same time. It's impossible right now. I mean, what is he thinking? Another marriage? What does she know about my kids?"

"You know, my mom married a guy named Curt and they were together from the time I was seven until I was 15," I said. "He didn't replace my Dad but he did things Dad couldn't do, like helped me with my Algebra and came to my school plays. Perhaps this woman and your kids will bond in a good way?"

Note to everyone: When your friend calls you needing to be talked off the ledge because her ex is getting re-married, you shouldn't suggest the new spouse might have some redeeming qualities.

"Are you fucking kidding me?!" She yelled. "She is an idiot and she thinks she's a better mother than I am. This is a nightmare!"

"OK, well when you calm down, try to say the mantra to yourself," I said. "Say it for yourself and no one else. Maybe it will help you. Screw them. Just worry about you right now."

The following morning, she called me on my way to work.

"So, after two hours of screaming and crying, I finally soaked in a bath and thought about what you were telling me," she said. "I couldn't remember exactly what the phrase was, so I thought about dip-shit and the future Mrs. dip-shit and said, 'I love you, thank you, I forgive you.' Was that was you were telling me to say?"

"Close enough," I said.

"Ok, so I said it. A few times. I kind of growled as I said it but I did it anyway. And then out of nowhere, I get an email from dip-shit today asking if we can get coffee because he wants to get my opinion about camps for the kids this summer," she said. "I was like, 'Huh?!' I don't think we've sat at the same table in three years."

"See?" I said.

"Well, I'm not holding my breath," she said. "He's probably trying to butter me up so he can side-swipe me in a few days but at least we can talk in person."

This woman and her ex-husband had been fighting for three years. He was moving on, and she was holding on.

Let it go!

I felt so relieved that my ex and I were not like most divorced couples.

"How long do I have to say that crap for it to really stick?" She asked.

"I don't know," I said. "Try doing it again tonight and see what happens."

"I don't know if I can because I'm going to the Bulls game. Unless it works if you do it when you're wasted?"

"I'm not sure," I said. "Give it a try and keep me posted."

⚜ ⚜ ⚜

A couple days later, Britt and I were driving to visit Grandma when a teenager using her phone cut me off on the highway.

"What is wrong with people?" I said, trying to avoid getting hit.

I love you, I'm sorry, please forgive me, thank you.

As I tried to avoid "Idiot number one" on my left, I looked to my right, and there was "Idiot number two" not watching where he was driving, also typing on his smartphone.

"Britt, when you grow up, promise me that you will never text and drive," I said.

"OK," he said, not looking up from his ipad.

"Why don't you put the ipad down and look for birds with me?" I asked.

I never thought I would be the kind of mom to allow her child to play video games in the car – until my mom moved to Wisconsin.

"No thanks," he said, engrossed in his game.

Spring was trying hard to make its presence known, but the rain and snow had frequented the landscape too often for any leaves or blooms to show their face. As a kid we used to drive to Wisconsin from Chicago all the time... Dad's family lived there most of my life.

My mind drifted from my Dad, to his Dad, John. Grandpa John was a radio announcer and broadcaster who moved to a farm in Wisconsin after he says the broadcasting world in Chicago "chewed him up and spit him out." Creatively, he was a genius, but the truth was, he was a terrible businessman. He started a television station in Chicago called WCIU because he felt every ethnicity should have a voice. He put bullfighters, wrestlers and Polish cooks on the air. He gave anyone a show. Even today, WCIU, or "Weigel Broadcasting", is known for its diversity.

John started every conversation with the same sentence: "What do you weigh these days?" Even when my father was a full-grown man with two kids, this was the most important morsel of information in John's eyes – whether his family members had gotten fat. I'm convinced this started me on a path of weight paranoia in my teens.

For some reason, I really was eager to win this man over when I was younger. Even when he cut my Dad off for seven years over an argument that took place at my Dad's high school reunion, I took a pen to paper to write John a heartfelt note. I was only a sophomore in college but I could see how torn up my father was over the fact they'd gone from talking everyday to complete silence. So I begged John to talk to his son. I closed the note with a simple sentence: "Even though you aren't speaking to my Dad right now, you are still my Grandpa and I for that, I still love you."

A few weeks later, I received the most evil note a man could write his 19-year-old granddaughter that ended with the line:

"Since Tim is no longer my son, it's impossible for you to be my granddaughter."

Ouch.

Obviously there was no love lost when John died a year after my father passed away.

I love you, I'm sorry, please forgive me, thank you.

I'd been doing my forgiveness chant every day, but the one person on my list I was having trouble with was Grandpa John.

"It is a choice to stay angry and bitter. You holding on to your grandfather's behavior is only holding *you* hostage, not anybody else." My friend John St. Augustine told me.

A stop sign jarred me back into present time. As I looked both ways before continuing, I was struck by the beauty of a hawk sitting on the fence next to the intersection.

"Britt! Look!" I yelled. My son put his game down and looked out the window.

"That's a Cooper's Hawk too," he said. My son, the budding ornithologist, could proudly list every hawk species that lived in the Midwest.

"OK, you know what, I want you to give me that ipad," I said, reaching for my device.

"Noooooooo!" He cried. A struggle ensued and I won.

"I want you to sit back and look for birds," I said.

"We won't see anymore," he pouted. "You've already seen them all. They're all gone."

"You have to trust. We are both going to sit back and trust and look for birds."

I turned up the radio, took a deep breath and tried to take my own advice.

A few minutes in, we passed by a barn that looks exactly like my Grandpa's old farm.

Just when I was starting to feel relaxed!

I noticed a sharp pain in my stomach. Just thinking about this man caused me physical harm.

Why can't I conquer this?

At that moment, I decided to muster up as much love as I could in my heart and pictured sending it to the ghost of my dead Grandpa. I put him right in front of me as I was driving, and rather than imagining I was hitting him with my car with a "Take that, you crabby son of a bitch!" I pictured a ball of light going from my heart into his.

I am not angry. I am sending unconditional love. I choose not to feel anger. I choose to feel love and forgiveness.

As I continued to breathe in and out, I was overwhelmed with a feeling of warmth. My eyes filled up with tears, and before I knew it, I was silently crying.

Love, forgiveness, gratitude.

After the initial swell of emotion, my heart rate started to stabilize. I felt calm and neutral. My stomach didn't hurt. I saw John's face and it actually looked tired and sad. I felt compassion for this man for the first time in my life.

People are only mean because they are afraid. Their fear turns into rage and their hateful behavior is simply their attempt to hide their insecurities.

Pay no attention to the scared asshole in the corner!

I wondered what kind of childhood my grandfather had to make him so scared, and then so mean.

I pictured John's face on a balloon and releasing it to the sky. I then did the same with every face from my "forgiveness" list.

I give it up to you, universe.

I drove in silence for a few moments, feeling complete peace.

And then,

"Oh my gosh Mom. *Look up*!!"

I looked up through the glass of our sunroof and saw a swarm of birds.

"Are those seagulls?" I asked.

"No Mom, those are hawks!" Britt screamed.

"Are you sure they aren't crows?" I asked.

"No Mom, seriously. Stop the car."

I tried to follow the birds with my eyes but there were too many to count. I decided to pull over in a parking lot so I wouldn't crash.

"Can you *believe* it?!" Britt gushed.

While at first I figured my son was having a spell of wishful thinking, I took a long hard look at the way these birds were flying. I've seen enough birds to know the difference between a seagull, a crow, a buzzard, an eagle and a hawk. A hawk has a certain stride in their glide – their wings are broad and majestic. Not only were these hawks flying above us, but I lost count at 40.

I never would have believed it had I not seen it with my own eyes.

"That is incredible!" I sighed. "Truly incredible."

I looked back at Britt and he was pointing his finger at the sky, trying to count the hawks. The expression on his face rivaled anything I'd ever seen, including the excitement of Christmas morning.

"I think there's 41," he said, his voice whispering with amazement. "Yes. 41."

We both sat there for a moment in silence, trying to absorb the miracle that had taken place. I had seen something I never would have believed to be possible.

And by sending love to the spirit of my Grandpa, I had done something that I never thought would be possible too.

"See what happens when you trust?" I said, still in shock at the view above.

See what happens when you send love instead of hate?

❧ ❧ ❧

CHAPTER SIXTEEN
SLOW DOWN AND ENJOY THE VIEW

Facebook Status:

Heard on Michigan Avenue: "Do you have plans tonight?" one girl asked another. "No. But I just found out that May is National Masturbation Month, so now I can celebrate in solitude."

⚜ ⚜ ⚜

A few days before day 40, I made an appointment with intuitive, Anne Emerson, to "re-pattern" my brain. She would do this over the phone.

"Walk me through what it is you'll be doing exactly," I said, wondering what I'd gotten myself into.

"You and I are going to talk, I'm going to listen and I'm going to write down what I hear you say that is an articulation of your blocks and your negative thoughts, which are kind of anchored in your unconscious that you don't even hear anymore," she explained. "I also can read under the surface. I'm just helping you do your job. I am the one who holds the flashlight so we can lift the rocks and look through the cracks. We're in the dark and I've got the flashlight, OK?"

An intuitive therapist! Cool!

"The unconscious is like a three-year-old having a tantrum," she continued. "It only deals in the most extreme form of language. Everything's either terrible or wonderful. Black or white. Good or bad. So when the unconscious 'sees' an experience that previously garnered a negative result, it can't tell if it felt like a pinprick or a sword. If it's even got a slight flavor of a past, unresolved traumatic issue, your unconscious goes immediately into defcon 5."

"So if I get an email from someone cancelling dinner plans, and I have a strong reaction, chances are it's because it's reminding me of my abandonment issues, and not that I'm totally pissed I'm missing out on sushi," I said.

"Exactly! Your body will react and shut down, and create experiences and responses that you needed to survive at a much earlier age. But these responses are no longer protectors. They have now become detriments. So we want to get in there and clear those babies out."

Yes! Let's clear those babies out!

"You go ahead and tell me what your blockages are, and I am going to be writing as you speak; and then I will pull out a one-sentence belief that you put into your system, because that's what you thought it needed to survive," Anne said. "Some of these beliefs might be inherited from Mommy and Daddy. I'll give you an example. I had the belief system that I couldn't have freedom and be in a relationship. I had the unconscious wiring that I couldn't be free and be myself and be in a relationship. When I processed through that I met my husband a month later. We've been married 17 years. It's really amazing."

I thought for a minute about what I wanted to focus on.

"I'm opening myself up to the possibility of loving again," I said. "I've been divorced a couple of years and I thought maybe I didn't want a relationship. But I think I'm ready, I just want to be sure I'm not repeating any of the old patterns. I want the next time to be different. I've always been the pursuer. So I've been saying to the universe, 'I'm ready to be pursued by someone I'm really attracted to.' I also want someone who is open to new experiences, who celebrates me and who excites me."

Do everything differently.

"I'm going to tell you some statements that I was hearing as you were talking," Anne said. "I heard you say, 'I don't trust men to come for me in love so I have to chase them down for a relationship. My fear of being abandoned is stronger and more real than any love and healing I receive from the divine. I'll just fall back into my old patterns with men. It's just a matter of time.'"

"Wow, those belief systems blow," I said.

"Yeah, we're gonna clear this crap out of here," she said. "But first, I need to ask you about the love relationship you had when you were 21?"

When I was 21?

As Anne posed the question, my mind took me back to a college boyfriend.

"I was with someone who actually pursued me so aggressively that he exhausted me into saying 'yes' to a date," I said. "I wasn't that interested in him. I grew to love him. We wound up dating for three years. But I was completely free and myself around him because I always thought, 'well, if he dumps me, that's OK.' We didn't have that intense chemistry that I had with other boyfriends. I felt safe with him, but not an intense connection. The ones I had chemistry with caused chaos and abandonment and drama."

"That was when you created the belief system that to be fearless in a relationship means there is no chemistry," she said. "If there is passion and you are 'in love,' then you have to be terrified of being abandoned. You created a distortion on passion."

A distortion on passion?

We pulled back more layers to find I had a belief system that you can't have a great career and a successful relationship because my parents and grandparents had all shown me it's either one or the other. She looked into certain behavioral patterns and helped me see why I had blocks in my self-esteem.

"We're going to rewire all of this and do a cognitive exercise where you say 'yes' to all of it. You are going to nod your head 'yes.' I want you to just let your head nod up and down, small or big sweeping motions, doesn't matter; I just want you to let your body surrender to the movement of 'yes.' Yes to the 'no' and yes to the 'yes.'"

I nodded my head as Anne talked.

I hope nobody is looking through my window right now.

"I want you to say this statement: 'I'm beautiful inside and out, and knowing this is true keeps me centered in what is real in love,'" she said.

I repeated this in my head and nodded "yes."

"I see who I am, appreciate what I create, and value what I bring to the table," she said.

Yes and yes.

"I am grateful that the divine is providing me the best opportunity for my evolution."

Yes. And yes.

"I am ready now to embrace the divine plan my spirit and soul have for me in this life."

Indeed.

"I say yes to co-creation, sex, cherished success, healthy boundaries, pleasure, travel, fun, marriage, now."

Yes. Yes. Yes. Yes. Yes. Yes. Yes. Yes; wait, marriage?

"I'm gonna say 'maybe' to the marriage," I told Anne.

"Your divine plan, however that looks," she said.

In that case, yes.

"Yes, God, to all of it. Thank you," she said.

She continued with some mantras and we finished up the session. I don't know exactly what she did to me but I felt like a weight had been lifted off of my shoulders.

"Now be sure to say this simple prayer each night: 'Yes, God, to all of it. Thank you.'"

Yes, God, to all of it. Thank you.

⚜ ⚜ ⚜

The following weekend I went walking with my friend, Liz. No matter how much I tried to change the subject, the conversation seemed to circle back to how I would choose the end of my 40-day "drought."

"Don't you have a male friend who could become a friend with benefits?" she asked.

"I don't think I could do that," I replied. "If I sleep with someone I'm like a golden retriever. I get very attached."

Do everything differently.

"What about Mr. East Coast?" Liz was one of the few friends I had who knew about him from day one. "I never would have guessed that would have turned into something."

"Yeah, me neither," I said.

⚜ ⚜ ⚜

When I first laid eyes on Mr. East Coast I didn't think he was my type.

"He's too much of a jock," I said to Liz as we spotted him across a crowded bar.

"His friends are all wasted too," she said. *"Next."*

He was so fit, I suspected he was a professional athlete. I watched him for a few minutes and studied his body language. When he laughed, he tipped his head back and used his entire body. When he listened he gave his subject complete focus. He looked at me and smiled. He held his gaze a few seconds too long. It was just enough to give me that funny feeling in the pit of my stomach.

I haven't felt that in ages.

"He's kind of cute," Liz said.

"I really like his laugh," I said.

He walked me along the ocean later that night and kissed me under the stars. The moment was right out of central casting: strong, attractive man, full moon, a passionate kiss. It made every hair on my body stand on end.

❧   ❧   ❧

"The thing I miss more than sex is getting kissed," I said to Liz as we continued our walk.

Everyone who is married or in a relationship for more than five years knows what it's like to have the kissing go by the wayside. By the time year five rolls around, kissing only happens when you're having "duty sex". When year 10 hits, duty sex becomes birthday sex and you're lucky if you even kiss at all.

Do everything differently…

A fabulous make-out session can be more satisfying than sex.

"Why not have East Coast man come here and you just compartmentalize it?" Liz suggested. "You have a history. You know his situation. You have chemistry."

"Because I think I deserve to be with someone who has the same feelings for me that I have for him," I said.

"Has he ever told you how he feels about you?" Liz asked.

"No," I admitted.

"Can't you find a friend who would at least kiss you at the end of your 40 days?" she asked.

I'd been so focused on the sex piece, I hadn't really thought about something like that.

"You know, that could be doable," I said.

"Only what happens if you start kissing and then you have trouble shutting things down?" she asked.

"Good point."

"Don't you have a vibrator?"

I'd been given a vibrator as a gift when I got divorced. It sits in my drawer unopened.

"Never been big into toys," I said.

"Well, how many days do you have left?" she asked.

"Not enough to find someone worthy of this kind of a title. I think I might have to just love myself."

"Nothing wrong with that," Liz laughed.

⚜   ⚜   ⚜

After work the next day, I decided to get a bikini wax; because as they say in the L'Oreal commercials, "I'm worth it!"

"Where have you been?" Marie, my bikini-waxer, asked as she gave me a hug.

"Not having sex, apparently," I said.

"You should do this regularly for *you*, with or without a man," she scolded, hitting my shoulder.

Love yourself, don't leave yourself.

I think women who pour hot wax around other women's vaginas should be paid six-figure salaries.

"The girls in the waiting area look so young," I said, staring at the ceiling. "Do you have a lot of young clients?"

"Yes. And you know, some of the younger ones will ask me, 'Do I look OK down there?' They're insecure about how their vagina is shaped or looks without hair."

"That's a shame," I said. "What do you say?"

"That's when I put my therapist hat on and tell them that every single person looks different down there, but a lot of them still don't believe me."

"Well if anyone would know, it's you," I laughed.

Riiiiiiiipppppppppppppppppp!

"Ow!"

"Sorry," she said, barely skipping a beat as she applied the next dollop of wax.

"So how's the book coming?" she asked.

"I'm doing a lot of reflecting right now on past relationships and why I chose certain people at different stages in my life. I can't believe I had such low standards when I was young. It really makes me sad for my teenaged self, you know?"

"Totally. I had this one boyfriend when I was in my early 20's, and I remember standing in front of him naked and he looked at me and said, 'You know, you'd be really hot if you had tits.'"

"Holy shit!" I said.

"I know, right?"

Riiiiiiiipppppppppppppppppp!

"Sorry," she said. "And of course I stayed with him too long and put up with so much of his crap, and it didn't work out anyway."

I looked at Marie's chest – and she had huge boobs.

"Did you get implants or something?" I asked.

"Oh no, these are real," she said. "They just sprouted all of a sudden, shortly after I dated that guy, actually."

"Too bad for him."

Riiiiiiipppppppppppppppp!

By now, the entire area below my waist was stinging.

"It's tough when you don't do this for awhile," I said, gritting my teeth.

"Sorry," she said, brushing loose pieces of wax away from my inner thigh. "So nobody in the dating world to speak of?"

"No," I said. "I went to dinner the other night with a guy who is divorced with four kids and he said to me, 'You know, you don't need a partner. You have your job and your son and your family and your friends and you don't have room for anyone.' And what I really think he was saying is 'You don't have time for me and my four kids.'"

"Well, that's probably true," she said.

Riiiiiiippppppppppppppp!

"Ahhhh!"

"Sorry. You OK?"

"Sure," I said, taking a deep breath.

"I mean, you don't want someone who thinks they need to fix you, and you sure as hell don't want to fix anybody else. That's codependent. But having someone you can share your life with, now that's something you want eventually, right?"

"I've been thinking about that more and more," I said.

"I'm in a really good place right now with my boyfriend," she said. "We're both divorced so we really focus on our communication. We just moved in together and it's going really well. I think we all deserve to have someone who wants to celebrate us, don't you?"

Marie grabbed a small mirror and handed it to me.

"Do people really inspect your work?" I asked, slightly horrified at the concept of looking at a magnified image of my newly bald, um, vagina.

"Sometimes," she said.

"No thanks," I said, handing the mirror back. "I trust you."

On day 40, my John of God roommate Amber and I got together to "celebrate" with an iced tea.

We sat outside on the first warm day of spring to compare notes.

"Have you had any physical reactions since you've been back?" I asked.

"Yes," she said. "Two years ago I was diagnosed with HPV and they said it was the cancer forming kind, and I was overdue for a checkup, so I got one when I came back. And they said the virus was gone."

"Gone? Did you ask to have it taken away in Toronto?"

"I asked for John of God to give me 'all that I can handle, for my highest good,'" she said.

"Wow. Any other physical changes?"

"I had all sorts of shit happened," she laughed. "My eyes got all red and swollen, and then my ankle was totally sore and I was limping for a little bit. So I'd say on the Tuesday or Wednesday after we got back I was a little overwhelmed. I actually got really scared. I had to remind myself that I had asked for this. I'm a meditator and I've seen some wild healers, but this kind of freaked me out."

"How do you feel now?" I asked.

"Amazing!" she said. "My eyes finally cleared up and my ankle, it's totally fine. I'd had problems with it for years but now it doesn't hurt at all. I'm so grateful."

"I can't believe I met John of God and couldn't ask my questions," I said.

"It's so funny because I see you as Super Woman, and Super Woman had a moment of weakness; and I was like, 'what?'" she laughed. "We all have our weak moments."

"I bet your boyfriend is glad the 40 days are behind us," I said.

"Absolutely!"

"I couldn't imagine laying next to someone without being intimate," I said.

"Usually exercise is my outlet and to not be allowed to do that, I really had to face all my fears and insecurities," she said. "All these emotions were coming up and I had no way to soothe myself. And then one time I woke up to my boyfriend sucking my left tit. I was like, "Get away from me! I'm only on day 23!"

"So what time are you having sex tomorrow?" I asked.

"As soon as possible!"

Lucky.

"How about you?" Amber asked. "How do you feel? Did John of God heal you?"

"Well, I know he did something," I said. "I want to do everything differently. Moving forward, how are you going to live differently?"

"I never want to be unconscious – unaware – again," she said. "I just want to live in a completely conscious world from now on. When we're a couple months out of this I don't want to get distracted and fall off the spiritual wagon."

"Anita Moorjani from the book, "Dying to be Me" had a near-death experience. True story: she had 24 cancerous tumors, some the size of lemons, and when she woke from her coma, all of her tumors were gone. She said that her experience was like ... if you are blind your whole life and then you are given the gift of sight – but then it's taken away – you might not be able to see anymore but you still won't forget what it feels like to see colors. So that's what this was like for me. I experienced something that I can't forget. Now I'm waiting for the love bath."

"Ask yourself 'What does love feel like?' Have you ever done that before?" Amber asked. "Just sit somewhere and open yourself up to it. It might take ten minutes. But you can feel it right in your heart. 'What does the love in the world feel like?'"

⚜ ⚜ ⚜

Day 41 finally arrived and there was no Knight in Shining Armor; no East Coast man knocking at my door. Just me, myself and I.

So that night I decided to fix myself up as though I were going on the most important date of my life. I pulled out a new razor, shaving cream, my favorite soap, and new shampoo and conditioner. Instead of racing through the process, I washed every curve and surface on my body with care, like I was handling a newborn baby. I even spent extra time on the parts that have given me angst, telling them how much I loved them.

I love you, c-section scar.

As I was drying off I reached for the spa lotion I'd been saving for that special occasion and held it over my legs. The lilac scent filled the air as I rubbed the silky texture into my skin. I opened my closet and picked out the black satin lingerie that I hadn't worn in months and put it on. I felt kind of silly looking at myself in the mirror, all gussied up.

Isn't this what you've been waiting for?

I'd finally been able to self-soothe, but when all was said and done, I didn't feel soothed at all.

I felt sad.

There I was, wearing nothing but my best lingerie and smelling like the spa at the Ritz Carlton, and I just wanted someone to hold me.

Hold yourself.

I pulled my knees to my chest and hugged myself for several minutes. While this helped a little, I still felt an intense void.

Why isn't this enough?

After a few minutes, I crawled into bed. I pictured the arms of God tucking me in and holding me until the loneliness dissolved. The glow of the nearly full moon came through my window as I took a deep breath. I soon realized I had a headache.

What's that smell?

The perfume-scented lotion was so pungent it was now making me feel nauseated. I got out of bed, removed my lingerie and got into the shower to wash off any remnants of my do-it-yourself spa treatment. As I was drying off, I saw a chunk of soap on the shower floor that was about the size of a nickel. I reached down to pick it up and as I turned it over, I couldn't believe my eyes. I was staring at a perfectly shaped heart.

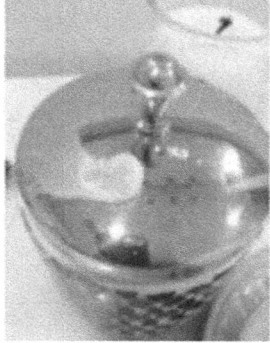

My Facebook friend, Kathy, sees hearts in all things: nature, food, carpet fragments. She often sends me pictures, reminding me that if I just keep an open mind, the hearts will show up. Now it was my turn to send *her* a picture.

It's amazing what you'll find when you look at things from a different perspective.

❧ ❧ ❧

Early the next morning, I got on the road and headed to visit my mom for the day to do some writing. I noticed the car in front of me was weaving slightly, so I tried to get out of the way. As I pulled around him to pass, I looked over and saw a mature, 60-something-year-ld man smoking pot.

Seriously?

This guy needed to "wake and bake" to get through his day.

Everyone self-soothes differently, I guess.

A few minutes later a car zoomed past me in a hurry. It had a vanity plate that read PICKLE.

Pickle?

Finally, a vanity plate that made me laugh.

After I arrived in Wisconsin I sat at the kitchen table looking out at the birds and the woods. I was able to write for hours. When I finally came up for air, I took a walk by the lake. As I strolled along the path I stopped in front a dock. I decided to sit down and take in the view. The heat of the sun soaked into my face, taking the chill out of the early spring breeze. I thought about Billy's words the last time we'd had dinner together.

"Why do women have such a hard time admitting they want to be in a partnership?"

I looked at the rocks under the water. Some of them sparkled like brilliant diamonds.

I trust you, God. Whatever is for my highest good, I trust you.

I watched several sticks and other debris float in the water over the rocks. And then one rock in particular caught my eye.

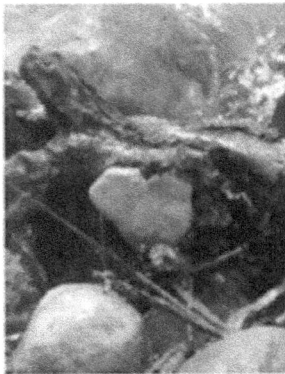

For the second day in a row I was seeing hearts.

After dinner, I got on the road. I left the music off and focused on the landscape. I saw a church from the highway with huge stained glass windows.

Maybe I should stop in?

I remembered Gail Thackray's words about how people left John of God and would start going back to their old ways. Within no time, their illnesses or problems would return.

No matter who you think will fix you; a healer, or therapist, or church – in the end, it's up to you to make those changes within.

My Mom has a saying, "No matter where you go, there you are."

I thought about my most recent conversation with Amber.

"Ask yourself 'What does love feel like?' Have you ever done that before? Just sit somewhere and open yourself up to it. It might take ten minutes. But you can feel it right in your heart. 'What does the love in the world feel like?'"

I took a deep breath and focused all of my energy into my heart. The image that came to mind was one of a steel door that almost looked medieval. I pictured the heavy pad lock being taken off as the large metal door creaked open. I saw a lot of dust and dark energy fly out of the door and all that was left was a deep red glow. At that moment, all the steel dissolved into thin air as the glow of my heart stayed strong. The light went from red to bright yellow, and finally it became white.

I then felt this overwhelming feeling of warm air as if it covered me like a blanket. I looked down on my arms and saw goosebumps. I also felt goosebumps at the top of my head. It seemed like I'd been touched by something bigger than myself, like I'd been washed with a feeling of love.

Is this what the love of the world feels like?

I looked ahead of me and the glow of a full moon was starting to show itself in the dusk sky. As I checked the rear-view mirror, there was a sunset covering the horizon with hues of red, purple and orange. Both the moon and the sun were in full view, and it was as if my future and my past were shining simultaneously. The bright moon was my hope – my dreams for what's to come. The setting sun was every step of the journey that led me to this moment.

Whether I was looking ahead or looking behind, the view was beautiful.

And your life is full, Jen.

I continued to admire the sky until a car cut in front of me going about 40 miles per hour. I got right up on his bumper so I could gently remind him of the rules of the road, but before I could flash my lights and honk in protest, I heard,

Slow down and enjoy the view.

Then I noticed the car's license plate – LOVEJOY.

Best. License plate. Ever.

I took my foot off the accelerator and laughed at the thought that God was showing me love comes in all forms.

Even in vanity plates!

I kept my eyes on the moon and did my best to enjoy the radiant view from all sides.

It was – for a lack of a better word – heavenly.

Thank you for showing me the next steps for my highest good and the highest good of all involved. No matter how it looks or shows up, help me trust it.

Yes God to all of it. Thank you.